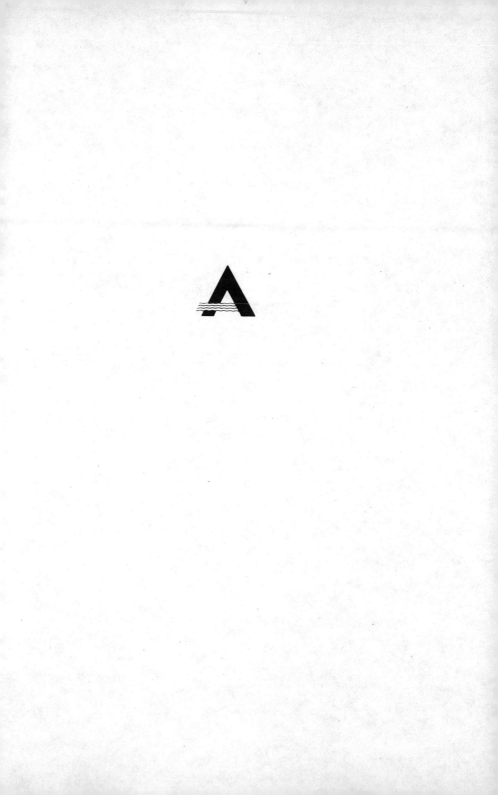

The Fertility Solution

The
Fertility Solution

....

*A Revolutionary Approach
to Reversing Infertility*

A. Toth, M.D.
with Jack Maguire

PRODUCED BY THE PHILIP LIEF GROUP

THE ATLANTIC MONTHLY PRESS
NEW YORK

Published simultaneously in Canada
Printed in the United States of America
FIRST EDITION

Library of Congress Cataloging-in-Publication Data

Toth, A.   The Fertility solution: a revolutionary approach to reversing
infertility / by A. Toth.—1st ed.
Includes index.
ISBN 0-87113-428-4
1. Infertility, Human—Chemotherapy. 2. Antibiotics. I. Title.
RC889.T68   1991   616.6'92061—dc20   90-42664

The Atlantic Monthly Press
19 Union Square West
New York, NY 10003

FIRST PRINTING

TO CONSTANCE

Contents

Chapter 1

....

New Hope for Reproductive Health

• Helen and Arthur[1] are childless despite unflagging efforts to conceive throughout a decade of marriage.

• David and Laura, the proud parents of twin boys born within nine months of their honeymoon, waited five years before trying to expand their family; today—two years later—they are still trying, in vain.

• Rhoda and Ed have endured the heartbreak of three miscarriages in as many years, but they are determined not to abandon the goal of producing a healthy baby.

Based on reported cases alone, almost 15 percent of adult Americans experience infertility. Despite medical advances in the treatment of infertility over the last two decades, that rate has not declined. In fact, most experts believe it has risen. Meanwhile, as the population of the United States has grown since 1970, the number of infertile couples has more than doubled. At present, an estimated 9 million individuals are affected by infertility.

Typically, couples like the ones mentioned above suffer silently through this epidemic for a long time before confronting

---

[1]Throughout this book, the names of all patients have been changed.

3

it. Once they finally do decide to seek help, most of them spend anxious months and thousands of dollars running in and out of specialists' offices and trying one fruitless treatment after another. It's an extreme exercise in pitting hope against frustration, perseverance against helplessness.

In fifteen years of practice as a pathologist and obstetrician-gynecologist at New York Hospital–Cornell Medical Center in New York City, I have examined and treated over forty thousand patients complaining of infertility. The majority of these patients have already invested years with other physicians by the time I see them. They are confused by the complicated and contradictory theories they have heard. They are exhausted by the invasive and costly tests and treatments they've undergone. And they are intimidated by all the advanced technology they've come to suspect may hold the only solution to their problem.

By contrast, what I offer my patients is a course of infertility treatment that is simple, painless, relatively inexpensive, and—most important—highly effective. Putting together what I have learned from my patients' histories, from my treatment of their cases, from my own research, and from dozens of other studies performed by my colleagues in the profession, I am convinced the fundamental cause of at least half of all infertility cases is common bacterial infections. Therefore, a high percentage of these infertility cases can be easily and safely reversed with the proper combination and dosage of antibiotics.

So far, the intensive antibiotic therapy for reproductive health problems that I recommend and administer has not been institutionalized across the country. Change moves slowly in any medical field and especially in a field as sensitive as infertility treatment. Many doctors are waiting for science to provide

4

them with more detailed information about the precise links between specific bacteria and specific infertility-related problems. Many laboratories used by doctors are not yet sophisticated enough to perform the intricate testing for bacteria that antibiotic therapy requires. Nevertheless, my antibiotic therapy is rapidly gaining attention and winning adherents. In the years to come, it promises to transform not only how medical science regards one of the most troublesome mysteries in biology but also how people in general look upon their own reproductive health care.

The revolutionary nature of antibiotic therapy in reversing infertility is most apparent in its phenomenal success rate. Overall, if no other cause of infertility besides infection can be documented, 60 percent of my infertility patients who receive this therapy go on to have trouble-free pregnancies that produce healthy babies—more than double the national average for other infertility clinics of comparable size and reputation. Even in cases where antibiotic therapy doesn't completely restore fertility, it functions as a critical first step in assisting other fertility therapies. Indeed, I have used it to alleviate many reproductive health problems that fall short of outright infertility, including premenstrual syndrome (PMS) and sexually transmitted diseases (STDs).

The essential rationale behind my therapy is mercifully easy to understand. The genital tract—male or female—can host hundreds of different kinds of bacteria. Basically, I believe that certain bacteria, several of which I have specifically identified, can turn pathogenic (that is, harmful) and cause infections that directly or indirectly contribute to a couple's inability to conceive a child or to a woman's ability to carry a child full term.

For men, the result of such a bacterial infection may appear in the form of a low sperm count, sluggish sperm activity, scar

5

tissue blocking sperm transmission, or physical destruction of the testes. For women, it may show up as cervicitis (causing stubborn vaginal discharge), endometritis (infection of the uterine lining), pelvic inflammatory disease (PID, which is characterized by extensive inflammation of any of the pelvic organs), a hormonal imbalance that upsets the ovarian cycle, or scar tissue blocking the fallopian tubes. Some bacterial infections betray themselves by causing the victim pain or discomfort. Others do their damage without generating any symptoms at all.

Sexual intercourse is the most well established mode of transmitting bacteria from one reproductive tract to another (although I have concluded bacteria can also be transmitted vertically—that is, from mother to child during the birthing process, an issue I will discuss in Chapter 3). In the context of sexual transmission, it is the female partner who generally suffers the most, thanks to the migrating capacity of sperm. Bacteria present in the seminal fluid prior to ejaculation—or present in the cervical or vaginal milieu prior to sexual intercourse—can attach themselves to sperm and "hitchhike" deep into the female partner's reproductive system, where they can colonize and jeopardize egg production, egg fertilization, and embryo implantation.

My task in reversing infertility-causing bacterial infections is multiphasic. First, I must look for clues that bacterial infection may have occurred in the history of the patient or the patient's sexual partners. Next, I must test appropriate cultures from both the patient and the patient's present partner to determine whether they harbor certain bacteria that are potentially harmful. Assuming I locate such bacteria, I must then treat both partners with a sufficiently strong antibiotic in a program of treatment lengthy enough to eradicate those bacteria. Finally, I must impose upon the couple a period of avoiding unprotected sexual intercourse until tests show that each partner's genital tract is completely clear of the suspect bacteria. At that point, I can be reasonably assured that their natural reproductive powers are on their way to restoring themselves. The high rate of post-therapy live births among my patients is testimony that my assurance is usually justified.

The Fertility Solution tells the story behind my theory about the origins of infertility; how I arrived at it, how I verified it, and how I developed my antibiotic therapy. It also demonstrates the steps I take to determine appropriate antibiotic therapies for different couples—therapies that succeed in either reversing their infertility or enabling them to derive benefit for the first time from other fertility therapies, including "fertility drug" treatments and assisted reproduction technologies such as artificial insemination and in vitro fertilization.

Before I begin this discussion, however, I must cite a few key facts about the general sociological background against which I have designed and applied my antibiotic therapy. Only then can the full value of the therapy be appreciated.

.... THE SILENT EPIDEMIC ....

As I indicated, the number of infertile couples in the United States has increased over twofold in the past twenty years. Today, the consensus of medical experts is that one in seven American men and women of childbearing age suffers from infertility. Either such infertile individuals have never been able to have a child, or they did produce one or more children before being rendered incapable of having another child. Why has the infertility rate continued to trend upward in the years since 1970? What bearing does this trend have on my theory about the infectious origin of reproductive health problems?

One factor responsible for the rising trend in infertility is that American men and women in general have become more sexually active, with—on a lifetime average—a greater number of sexual partners. This situation has fueled a significant spread of STDs—including, besides the well-known gonorrheal and syphilitic infections, the lesser-known infections caused by chlamydia and countless other pathogenic bacteria. Many of these infections, well known or lesser known, thrive unchecked in the victim's reproductive system because they are asymptomatic. They may not be detected until the victim, or the victim's partner, confronts the fact that he or she is unable to produce a child.

To a large extent, the introduction of convenient, reliable, and widely available birth control methods in the mid-1960s ushered in the era of sexual freedom, but some of those birth control methods came with enormous hidden costs. Aside from making a woman mistakenly believe that she was safe having frequent sex with any number of different partners, their particular operation or design (as I shall discuss later) allowed bacterial infections to penetrate farther into the user's reproductive system than they otherwise might have been able to go. I'll discuss such tragic side effects in more detail in Chapter 2.

Besides the ongoing sexual revolution and its attendant spread of disease, the other main factor contributing to the rising incidence of infertility in recent years has been the increasing trend among women to put off having a child until a later age. Their reasons are excellent: they want to wait until they've had a greater opportunity to enjoy freedom from parenting, until their relationship with their partner is more secure, until their career is more firmly established, until they can better afford the expenses associated with child rearing, or until they feel mature enough to be the nurturing kind of parent they want to be. Unfortunately, their timing is not as excellent as their reasoning.

The age bracket within which it is best for the average woman to bear a child is twenty to twenty-six. After the age of twenty-six, a woman's reproductive system begins to lose some of its efficiency and, therefore, its fertility. Today, according to the Office of Population Research at Princeton University, 25 percent of married women under the age of thirty have never had a baby by choice, compared with only 12 percent in the mid-1960s. While nine out of ten women between the ages of twenty and twenty-six are fully capable of producing a baby, the odds diminish to one out of four by the time a woman is thirty-five years old and to one out of five by the time she is forty.

In addition to suffering an inevitable natural weakening of her reproductive powers, the aging woman may be allowing an asymptomatic bacterial infection to cause increasing damage to her genital tract, to the point where she actually experiences what many doctors will diagnose as premature menopause. In my own practice, I have encountered numerous examples of this kind of bacterial damage. Fortunately, I have also been able many times to reverse the damage and restore the victim's fertility with antibiotic therapy.

9

.... THE PATH TO DISCOVERY ....

Now that I have summarized critical sociological elements relevant to infertility, I want to share with you some aspects of my personal background that led me to establish the connection between bacterial infections and infertility. It is my hope that this brief review will give you a better sense not only of the science behind this book but also of the scientist behind this book.

My fascination with the mysteries of reproductive health began when I was fifteen years old and still living in my native Hungary. My father, himself an obstetrician and gynecologist, took me into his laboratory and showed me a strange-looking tissue from the human uterus that he called *fasciculus cervico angularis*. He went on to take his discovery before a scientific audience and was ridiculed because no other anatomist had ever found the structure through dissection. A year later he died of Hodgkin's disease, which in those days was incurable. This sequence of events had a profound influence on me, leaving me with an overwhelming ambition to excel in medical science and a specific anatomical mystery to solve.

That ambition and that mystery carried me through six years of medical school in Hungary, a year of medical service in Austria, and after immigrating to the United States, four more years of studying pathology, including histology, cytology, and clinical chemistry, at Mount Sinai Hospital in New York City. It was during these last four years of study that I was finally able to locate the uterine structure my father had shown me long ago.

Dissecting scores of uteri, I photographed the *fasciculus cer-*

10

vico angularis using conventional cameras and the electron microscope. Then I published two papers crediting my father's work that verified its existence. The next step was to learn the function of this unusual structure. To do this, I had to become a clinician and treat living people, and so I embarked on a residency program in obstetrics and gynecology at the New York Hospital–Cornell Medical Center in New York City.

It was at the end of this residency that an extraordinary opportunity presented itself. Dr. John MacLeod, a world-famous expert in sperm analysis and the treatment of male infertility, was about to retire, and he wanted me to take over his laboratory at New York Hospital. Accepting this challenge meant postponing indefinitely my studies of the function of the *fasciculus cervico angularis,* but, reassured I could continue to see female patients one day a week in my private office, I accepted.

The years since then have made me enormously glad I accepted that position. I believe that combining my training as a pathologist and experience as an obstetrician and gynecologist with expertise in semen analysis and male-related reproductive health problems has given me a uniquely comprehensive perspective on infertility. I have brought this perspective to numerous studies designed to reveal how bacterial infections compromise a couple's reproductive health, and here's what those studies have shown:

Certain bacteria in human semen can adversely affect the shape and motility of sperm. Infections of this nature can be cured with antibiotic therapy, resulting in a return of well-formed and well-functioning sperm.

In November 1977 Christine Swenson, a microbiologist, came to my laboratory for a professional consultation. I re-

11

member the date well because this short meeting was the first in a chain of events that led me to practice antibiotic therapy as I do today. Swenson was then preparing her doctoral thesis on mycoplasma, a bacterium known to cause infections in the genital tract. Some authorities had alleged that these infections might lead to infertility, but no extensive research had yet been done. I agreed to collaborate with her on an experiment to test whether the presence of mycoplasma could be easily identified and treated.

From electron microscope photographs, we knew mycoplasma could attach themselves to the tail, midpiece, or head of the spermatozoon. Most often, they bond to the tail, where they appear as little beads and cause the tail itself to coil. Our experiment involved testing semen samples from one hundred men. Swenson cultured specimens for the organism while I, working independently and unaware of her findings, studied slides of the specimens under a microscope.

Whenever I found an excess number of spermatozoa with coiled tail segments or fine beads attached to them, I postulated that Swenson's culture report would be positive. After the one hundredth specimen had been run, her culture results and my guesses were compared. It turned out my predictions were correct in 75 percent of the cases.

After we published our findings in the November 1978 edition of *Fertility and Sterility,* the journal of the American Fertility Society, we decided to treat a group of patients to see how their mycoplasmal infections would respond to antibiotic therapy. We began by asking both the patients and their partners to take tetracycline orally four times a day for a month. This therapy achieved a disappointingly low cure rate of 54 percent.

We repeated the experiment using a newer, broader-spectrum antibiotic drug, Vibramycin, with a treatment regimen of two doses a day. This time, our cure rate was 80 percent. After therapy, the cured patients' spermatazoa were more streamlined in appearance and were moving much faster, so it was logical to conclude that the Vibramycin had removed virtually the entire bacterial load they had been carrying. It was also logical to conjecture from all our studies to date that mycoplasma may be capable of interfering with the infected male's fertility simply by reducing the speed and forward movement of the spermatozoa.

At that time, we temporarily attributed all the favorable changes we observed in semen quality after antibiotic therapy to the eradication of one organism: mycoplasma. We quickly came to realize, however, that the type of broad-spectrum antibiotics we were using against mycoplasma could also work against other, as yet unobserved and unidentified bacteria that were also harmful.

In the years following this series of experiments, I increased the Vibramycin dosage in my therapy for mycoplasmal infections, and I complemented this treatment with three additional weeks of erythromycin. The result was a 97-percent success rate. In addition, I established that chlamydia and certain anaerobic bacteria can adversely affect spermatozoa and can be effectively treated with appropriate antibiotic therapy. I'm sure future studies will reveal other bacteria that are harmful as well, some of which my therapy may already be destroying.

One important development that arose from those early studies of mycoplasma was their influence on many other doctors across the nation. Although the dosages I recommended were exceptionally high and long lasting according to the standards set by the *Physicians' Desk Reference,* these doctors began to prescribe them in their own practices. And so a movement began.

Today, my antibiotic therapy remains experimental by definition even though it is steadily becoming more and more routine in the field of reproductive health care. My answer to those doctors who continue to question the comparatively high and long-lasting dosages is this: once you accept the facts that harmful bacteria exist, that they may adversely affect fertility, that they can be eradicated only by high and long-lasting antibiotic dosages, and that patients rarely suffer any negative side effects from such dosages, then you must be consistent as well as conscientious and treat harmful bacterial infections to the point of cure.

Men whose seminal fluid is infected with harmful bacteria are far more likely to be infertile than are men whose seminal fluid is not so infected.

By the end of 1980, I had completed a two-year study involving 430 randomly selected married male patients. They were divided into five groups according to their history:

- *Group A*—fertile men whose wives had achieved two or more pregnancies within two months of trial and were currently pregnant

- *Group B*—men from primarily (that is, no child) or secondarily (that is, no child after one or more children) infertile marriages with no history of genital-tract infection

- *Group C*—men from primarily or secondarily infertile marriages with a history of nonspecific urethritis (inflammation of the urethra, a fairly common male complaint) during the last ten years

- *Group D*—men from primarily or secondarily infertile marriages with a history of prostatitis (inflammation of the prostate gland, a less common, more serious male complaint) during the last ten years

- *Group E*—men from primarily or secondarily infertile marriages with a history of treated gonorrhea (an even more serious reproductive health problem) during the last ten years

Group A, the fertile group, was the control for the study, and men in this group had the least number of premarital sexual contacts among all five groups. Of the four infertile groups, group B men had the least number of premarital sexual contacts; group E, the most. I cultured semen specimens from each volunteer for bacterial isolates. The fewest isolates were found in specimens from group A men. Among the four other groups, specimens from group B men had the least amount of bacterial isolate; specimens from group E men, the most (including a high frequency of mycoplasmal and anaerobic bacteria).

The implication of these results is clear. Asymptomatic bacteria can develop and multiply in a man's seminal fluid after he has had a clinically symptomatic or asymptomatic genital-tract infection, and these bacteria can reduce the man's fertility.

Sperm play an active role in transmitting potentially harmful bacteria throughout a woman's genital tract.

The next logical step in my investigation of the link between bacterial infections and infertility was to prove my theory that a bacterially contaminated man could infect his partner through sexual intercourse—or, more accurately, through exposure to his seminal fluid. Knowing that bacteria could attach themselves to spermatozoa, I was convinced that they could travel wherever the spermatozoa might go and, thus, that they could infect a woman's reproductive system as far up as the fallopian tubes and ovaries.

In 1982, after much creative thought, I set about replicating, under laboratory conditions, the sperm's journey through a woman's cervix, which functions as a gateway between the vagina and the uterus. Cervical mucus has always been considered an effective mechanical and immunological barrier between the bacterial flora of the vagina and the upper genital tract. Therefore, I wanted to create a milieu of cervical mucus through which contaminated sperm could swim so I could see whether the same bacteria that attached to the sperm before their journey were newly present in the cervical fluid after their journey.

First, I drew cervical mucus into sterilized microhematocrit tubes that measured 75 millimeters in length with a diameter of 1.1 millimeter. Then, I placed each filled tube upright in a small, shallow well of bacteria-laden seminal fluid, obtained from samples donated by patients visiting my laboratory for infertility consultation. To monitor the time it took the sperm to migrate throughout the microhematocrit tubes, I placed a mucus-filled tube under a microscope and immersed one end of the tube in semen.

In about an hour, the "far" end of the microhematocrit tube under the microscope showed that a significant number of sperm had arrived, so I terminated the experiment. I broke off the upper third of each microhematocrit tube and cultured the mucus inside.

In every tube that had been submerged in semen containing sperm, all bacteria that had originally been present in the semen (including anaerobic bacteria) could be found in the upper third of the cervical mucus, together with motile sperm. By design, I had included in the experiment some semen samples containing bacteria but no sperm, and in the upper third of the cervical mucus corresponding to these semen samples, no bacterial migration could be detected.

Thus, I established strong evidence that bacteria-contaminated sperm can carry infection into a woman's upper genital tract. My experiment also suggests that bacteria-free sperm are capable of transporting bacteria from a woman's vagina into the upper genital tract, thus enabling resident bacteria to bypass the natural barrier to "unassisted" bacteria created by the cervical milieu.

Bacterial infections can lead to infertility. The odds of infertility are dramatically reduced if an infected couple undergoes antibiotic therapy.

After completing all the studies I've described so far (as well as other studies that supported my initial findings), I still needed to forge the final links between bacterial infection and infertility and between antibiotic therapy and the reversal of infertility. I did this in 1983, when I completed a three-year follow-up study comparing the pregnancy rates of two different groups of women:

1. Women whose husbands' mycoplasma infections were successfully eradicated by antibiotic treatment, as demonstrated by a negative post-therapy semen culture

2. Women whose husbands' mycoplasma infections were not successfully eradicated by antibiotic treatment, as indi-

cated by the persistent presence of mycoplasma bacteria in
their post-therapy cultures

There were 161 couples in the study. All of them—husbands
and wives—took 100 milligrams of doxycycline twice a day for
four weeks, and in 129 cases (80 percent of the couples), the
husband's mycoplasma infection was successfully eradicated.
Among these 129 couples, 60 percent went on to experience a
successful pregnancy, a dramatic contrast to the 5-percent pregnancy rate among the other 32 couples in the study (that is,
those in which a husband's infection was not eradicated).

The results of this study were even more impressive than I
thought they would be. On March 3, 1983, they were published in the *New England Journal of Medicine* and reported
in the *New York Times* and various other newspapers via Associated Press; and ever since then, more and more specialists
and infertile couples have turned to antibiotic therapy to prevent bacterial infections from resulting in genital-tract damage. Nevertheless, my work is far from over. Antibiotic
therapy deserves to receive much more attention—not just because it has the capacity to eradicate infections, but—much
more importantly—because it has the capacity to prevent
them.

This book will show you how antibiotic therapy has worked
for others, and it will empower you to make better, more informed decisions about your own reproductive health care. My
personal hope is that the information presented here will also
inspire you to anticipate problems you or your loved ones may
face, and to take positive action to keep such problems from
happening in the first place.

Chapter 2

....

The Causes of Infertility:
Facts and Fallacies

Under exceptional and relentless pressure from all quarters of society to find a cure for infertility and to ensure the well-being of unborn children, medical science has learned a great deal in the past two centuries about human reproduction. For the most part, however, the subject remains a miraculous mystery.

We know many of the basic mechanisms that assist conception, pregnancy, and birth but very few of the fine points regarding how and why these mechanisms function the way they do. In the absence of such knowledge, we operate on theories. By following these theories, we can frequently influence reproductive processes to function the way we want them to. Nevertheless, we seldom know for certain how or why this happens.

At best, any therapy or procedure to facilitate healthy reproduction is imprecise and partial, although it may turn out to be successful. Given the incredible intricacy of the natural reproductive process, there is no such thing as a sure cure when it malfunctions. There are only degrees to which certain problems can be minimized. Most infertility patients assume modern science has more answers than, in fact, it does. Essentially, the best that doctors can offer their infertility patients is informed strategies for navigating their way through largely unknown and unpredictable territory.

Before I go into specific detail about how antibiotic therapy has helped my patients reach their goals, I'd like to set some parameters for that discussion. This chapter will briefly explore what we can say, with some certainty, about what makes a couple infertile. It will also look into the more widespread and damaging misconceptions about infertility I've encountered in talking with my patients. These discussions will establish the basic rationale behind my theory that at least 50 percent of infertility problems are due to bacterial infection.

WHAT DOES *INFERTILE* .... MEAN? ....

Definitions of infertility vary greatly even within the medical profession. According to William D. Mosher of the National Centre for Health Statistics, which sets the standard for many medical specialists, a couple is considered infertile "if they are not surgically sterile [that is, rendered sterile by a surgical operation] and have not been able to conceive after a year or more of unprotected intercourse."

I define infertility much more strictly, adding two other conditions. First, I don't consider a couple fertile unless the female partner has been able to carry a baby full term to a live birth. Second, I don't consider a couple fertile unless the baby they produce is healthy—that is, not underdeveloped, colicky, or unusually vulnerable to infectious illnesses.

Many doctors would agree with my first additional condition. Very few would extend their definition of infertility to include my second additional condition. Be that as it may, I believe human reproductive systems—male and female—are wondrously well designed to produce healthy babies. If, instead, a couple produces a baby whose health has been adversely affected by the poor quality or shortened duration of the pregnancy, then I would say without hesitation that the couple has an infertility problem—and one that might easily worsen with time.

For fourteen years, I continued to be a practicing obstetrician despite strong temptations to devote myself entirely to my research and therapy in reproductive health. I retained my role as an obstetrician because I insisted on superintending the final results of that research and therapy. In other words, I felt my mission to reverse a couple's infertility was not complete until I had done everything I could to deliver a healthy baby on or near the date he or she was due to be born. In most of my cases, thankfully, that is what happens.

There is yet another aspect to the basic distinction between fertility and infertility—an aspect to which I referred in Chapter 1. A couple can be either *primarily* infertile or *secondarily* infertile. In cases of primary infertility, the couple has never been able to conceive (or, by my definition, produce) a child. In cases of secondary infertility, a couple has managed to conceive—or produce—one or more children in the past but no longer appears capable of doing so (again, after a year or more of unprotected intercourse).

As I will explain in more detail later, many cases of secondary infertility in particular can be attributed to bacterial infection. The logic behind such a pattern is easy to follow. Harmful bacteria first gain entry into the female partner's genital tract at the time of her previous successful conception.

The pregnancy resulting from that conception does produce a live baby, but it's quite likely the pregnancy itself is troubled, or the delivery is premature, or the baby is somewhat sickly. By the time the couple tries for another pregnancy, the bacterial infection in the woman's genital tract has spread, and the damage is sufficient to prevent conception or cause a miscarriage.

So far, I have discussed only the infertile *couple.* I prefer to define fertility or infertility in terms of couples rather than individuals because it is only in the context of the couple that an individual demonstrates his or her fertility or infertility. Someone who is infertile with one partner may be fertile with another partner for reasons medical science may not be able to ascertain.

Of course, there are specifically male-related and female-related infertility problems that can work singly or in tandem to prevent a couple from having a child. In subsequent chapters of this book, I'll examine these major infertility problems in terms of the different therapies used to address them, concentrating mainly on antibiotic treatment. But for now, let me simply identify these problems.

Problems Associated with Infertility: Female (arranged, approximately, from most common to least common)

- *Damaged fallopian tubes*—blockage or scarring prevents the egg and sperm from uniting or prevents the united egg and sperm from descending to the uterus for maturation (resulting in an ectopic pregnancy).

- *Abnormal ovulation*—the egg-production cycle is not functioning normally due to hormonal deficiencies or imbalances.

24

- *Pelvic inflammatory disease* (**PID**)—this umbrella term refers to an inflammation of any of the pelvic organs, including the reproductive organs, which can impede their ability to foster conception or support a pregnancy.

- *Endometriosis*—the uterine lining (or endometrium) grows outside the uterus, resulting in excess bleeding, blockage, or scarring in the surrounding reproductive structures, which can interfere with conception or pregnancy.

- *Damaged ovaries*—scarring prevents proper egg development, fertilization, or release.

- *Hostile cervical mucus*—excess acidity or antibodies in the milieu of the cervix (situated between the vagina and the uterus) kills the sperm before they can reach the eggs.

- *Incidental causes*—this category includes damage inflicted on any part of the reproductive system by a major abdominal disease, surgery, therapy (such as chemotherapy), tumor (such as fibroid tumor), physical trauma, or drug exposure.

Problems Associated with Infertility: Male (arranged, approximately, from most common to least common)

- *Idiopathic low sperm count* (unknown cause of a reduced sperm count)—this is the most commonly observed fertility abnormality in the male, probably caused by an unknown intrauterine factor that adversely affected the development of the testes during the male's embryonic life. Unfortunately, if bacterial cultures are negative, and the hormones are normal, and there is no varicocele, this particular abnormality resists all currently available treatments.

- *Dilated veins around the testicle*—this condition, known as varicocele, increases the temperature in the scrotum, which can result in fewer sperm as well as malformed or malfunctioning sperm (that is, poor swimmers).

- *Damaged sperm ducts*—blockage or scarring in the sperm ducts (or vas deferens) prevents the sperm from reaching the seminal fluid.

- *Hormone deficiency*—there is an insufficient or too-erratic release of the hormones that stimulate sperm production.

- *Impotence*—the man is unable to ejaculate inside the vagina due to disease (such as hardening of the arteries, high blood pressure, diabetes, or kidney disease), environmental factors (such as substance abuse or certain medication regimens), or psychological factors (such as performance anxiety or premature ejaculation).

- *Sperm antibodies*—in rare cases (for example, among a small fraction of men who have undergone vasectomy reversals), the immune system develops antibodies to the sperm that kill the sperm as soon as they are produced.

- *Incidental causes*—this category includes any damage caused by a major abdominal disease, surgery, therapy (such as chemotherapy), tumor, drug exposure, or physical trauma.

THE ROLE OF BACTERIAL
.... INFECTION ....

I did not single out bacterial infection as a problem leading to infertility in either of the above lists. This is because I'm convinced bacterial infection is a probable underlying or aggravating cause of virtually all these problems. This is not to say a bacterial infection by itself isn't a problem that can lead to infertility—the rest of the book will make this clear.

In a woman, harmful bacteria can give rise to disasters anywhere in the genital tract. They can form adhesions that block or scar the fallopian tubes and/or the ovaries. They can spur the development of endometriosis or PID. They can offset natural hormone cycles. And they can trigger adverse chemical changes in the cervical mucus.

In a man, the same kinds of harmful bacteria (and, no doubt, others we haven't yet isolated) are similarly far-reaching. They can have a directly negative impact on the volume, morphology, or motility of the sperm wherever the sperm may go. They can also have an indirectly negative impact on sperm production by damaging the testicles. And they can generate adhesions that block or scar the sperm ducts.

Because bacteria are so small, so elusive, and so often asymptomatic, it is extremely difficult to prove the exact nature of their contribution to any given case of infertility. That is why most lists of problems leading to infertility—like the two lists above—are organized according to grosser, more observable phenomena that manifestly distinguish one particular infertility case from another. The special challenge of my career has been not just to accumulate evidence that bacterial infection does, in fact, lie at the root of most infertility problems but to identify and classify the specific bacteria that can be troublesome.

Among all the bacteria that can be found in human reproductive systems, mycoplasma, chlamydia, and certain anaerobic bacteria are potentially harmful. How did I go about determining this? Basically, I approached the problem by creating good-guy versus bad-guy criteria for judging individual bacteria.

Good guys are any bacteria I can determine were present in a woman's genital tract during two successful reproductive processes (that is, from conception to birth on two different occasions). Given such circumstances, I can reasonably assume the bacteria in question are not likely to cause any interference with reproductive health. I insist on two successful reproductive processes to reduce the odds that I may be dealing with a sample from a woman who is, in fact, developing secondary infertility.

Bad guys, by contrast, are any bacteria that appear in the genital tracts of only those women who have had reproductive problems—for example, conception hasn't occurred, or there was a miscarriage, or there was an overly long period of labor. Through meticulous record keeping and repeated studies of cultures from couples whose reproductive histories fit either the former or the latter category, I have been able to identify mycoplasma, chlamydia, and certain anaerobic bacteria as bad guys.

My work is far from over. Besides these three unmasked bad guys, there are hundreds of bacteria for which I'm not (and, to my knowledge, no one else is) yet able to test, including other anaerobes, aerobes, viruses, yeasts, and parasites.

Frankly, anaerobes interest me the most of all these types of bacteria because, like the worst villains in any scenario, they are so charismatic. According to what science has been able to discover to date, not only do anaerobes possess all sorts of capacities to toy unpredictably with the human immune system, but they can also act as co-culprits with other bacteria.

And they are numerous. The ratio between anaerobic bacteria and other bacteria in the average person's genital tract is somewhere between ten to one and twenty to one. This fact more than any other indicates that anaerobic bacteria are the most important ones for me to study in order to isolate any more bad guys. Meanwhile, it's only logical to assume my broad-spectrum antibiotic therapy is killing some of these unknown villains at the same time it is killing the known ones.

When I culture specimens from a couple suffering from infertility and find suspect bacteria in both the male and the female samples, there is always at least one harmful kind of bacterium that both samples have in common. This pattern further corroborates my theory that bacterial infections are sexually transmitted. In most cases of sexual transmission (as I discussed in Chapter 1), the male sperm carries the harmful bacteria into the female genital tract, although it's also possible, to a lesser degree, for a bacterially contaminated woman to infect her bacteria-free male sex partner.

Such officially recognized STDs as gonorrhea and syphilis can spur the infectious activity of other harmful bacteria, like mycoplasma, chlamydia, and certain anaerobes, that are already present but dormant in a person's genital tract. They can also bring these other harmful bacteria with them. During the latter half of the 1980s, chlamydia finally earned widespread acknowledgment as a full-fledged STD. In my opinion, all bacterial infections should be officially recognized as STDs, an issue I'll pursue further in Chapters 5 and 6.

Another way in which bacteria can spread deep into a woman's genital tract (that is, beyond the cervix into the uterus, fallopian tubes, and ovaries) is through the use of certain types of birth control methods. Intrauterine devices (IUDs) offer the greatest potential risk.

The IUD prevents pregnancy by triggering an inflammation inside the uterus, which makes it impossible for an embryo to implant itself there. The user's normal hormonal cycle continues unchanged, however. The cervix undergoes its monthly estrogen-dominated phase, in which the mucus is favorable for sperm migration, and the sperm have no barrier to prevent them—along with any harmful bacteria they may be carrying—from traveling into the woman's upper genital tract. In addition, sperm can penetrate the cervix during the actual menstrual bleeding, and the bleeding time is typically much longer for IUD users. All these factors put together could well explain the marked increase in the rate of PID and other reproductive health problems among IUD users.

Birth control pills are somewhat safer when it comes to avoiding bacterial infection. The pill disrupts the normal hormonal cycle, thus creating a cervical mucus that is sticky and unfavorable to sperm. Nevertheless, pill users are vulnerable to sperm migration—and, hence, the spread of bacterial infection—beyond the cervix during their menstrual bleeding time.

The ideal birth control method for avoiding the risk of bacterial infection is the condom. When they use a condom, both partners are relatively safe from any contact with foreign body fluids that are bacteria-infected. Failing condom use, the female partner can protect herself by using a barrier-type device (like a diaphragm) for birth control.

COMMON FALLACIES ABOUT
.... INFERTILITY ....

No medical condition provokes in its sufferers quite such a complicated mixture of anger, fear, shame, guilt, and hysteria as infertility. It is little wonder, therefore, that so many myths have arisen regarding the causes and cures of infertility—myths that presumably help infertile individuals vent their frustration, shield their embarrassment, assign blame, or simply account for the unaccountable.

Before moving on to examine in more detail what I believe is a woefully underacknowledged truth about infertility—that is, the major role bacterial infection can play—let me briefly expose the major fallacies associated with infertility, based on what many of my patients have said to me.

The female partner is usually responsible for a couple's infertility.

This is the most prevalent of all myths having to do with infertility. As statistics now stand, the two genders are equally responsible. About 35 percent of infertility cases in America are due to female-related problems, about 35 percent are due to male-related problems, about 20 percent are due to a combination of male- and female-related problems, and about 10 percent are inexplicable.

Given my belief that the majority of infertility cases originate in bacterial infection, and given my belief that sperm are the major vehicles for sexually transmitting such infections, I'd be inclined to say the male partner is usually responsible for a couple's infertility. I prefer, however, to treat all cases of infertility as a couple's—and not an individual's—problem and responsibility.

The myth that the female partner is usually responsible for a couple's infertility—which, to my mind, is the most damaging of all infertility myths—can be attributed almost entirely to sexism. For centuries, male-dominated medical science has insisted that women carry the burden of making reproduction work. Not only have men decided that making children is what a woman does, but they've also maintained a willful blindness toward the possibility that their ability to impregnate a woman successfully may be just as fragile as a woman's ability to achieve a successful pregnancy.

Women in developed nations are expected to perform the yearly ritual of going to a gynecologist (usually male) for a checkup. It may be a nuisance, it may be embarrassing, but it's something that has to be done. But how often do you hear men saying to each other, "What did your urologist say the last time you saw him [or her!]?" or "Can you give me the name of a good urologist?" or "I'm considering changing urologists."

I've never overheard such a conversation among men, although I frequently overhear the equivalent among women about their gynecologists. Until I do routinely hear men exchanging such remarks, I won't be satisfied that male partners are assuming the responsibility they should for the reproductive health of the couple.

Psychological problems are a major cause of infertility.
In fact, psychological problems are seldom a cause of infertil-

ity, although they can frequently be a serious *effect* of infertility. While it is true that cortical events (that is, strong emotions, such as depression) are capable of causing changes in male or female hormonal levels that can, in turn, adversely influence the reproductive system, this situation is very rare. People who have been in prison for years may suffer "psychologically induced" infertility, but under less extreme circumstances, it's highly unlikely such a thing will happen.

Certainly, psychological problems can have a negative impact on spontaneous sexual performance, often resulting in fewer instances of sexual intercourse than the affected man or woman might otherwise have. But the times when they do have sexual intercourse are not at all likely to be compromised by any infertility problems of a psychological nature.

It is not true that "just getting away from it all for a while" enhances a person's—or a couple's—chances of conceiving. What it does enhance are the chances that the couple will engage in sexual intercourse more frequently, which can be beneficial if the couple is otherwise having sexual intercourse only two or three times a month.

It does sometimes happen that couples who are unable to conceive and who finally decide to adopt a child do, in fact, conceive shortly after the adoption. This is not because a change in certain psychological factors has rendered conception possible, however. It is probably because the couple had been undergoing therapy for a long time to reverse infertility, and that therapy finally paid off. Otherwise, as far as science is concerned, it's simply fortuitous.

Infertility is a frequent aftereffect of abortion or rape.
I've had many patients who believe the physical or emotional trauma of an abortion or a rape has rendered them

infertile. Some women who have had an abortion believe God is punishing them by not letting them have another baby. Scientifically speaking, there is no evidence that an abortion or a rape will adversely affect one's fertility any more than a miscarriage or an act of consensual intercourse will, unless the abortion or rape involves some gross structural damage to the reproductive system.

Any conception, whether it occurs via rape or consensual intercourse can, of course, spread deleterious bacteria through the woman's genital tract. In the case of an abortion, especially if the woman has never given birth to a child or has previously given birth to only one child, secondary infertility may be the result of such an infection, but it will remain undetected until a subsequent attempt at pregnancy. The chances are high that any such condition can be reversed with the help of antibiotic therapy at that later date. In the case of rape, the victim may have been infected with bacteria-laden sperm, but this, too, can be treated.

Infertility has a negative impact on sexual performance or enjoyment.

There is no reason that an asymptomatic infertility condition should have any effect on one's sexual performance or enjoyment, including a woman's ability to have an orgasm or a man's ability to ejaculate. In cases where an infection in the male or female partner's genital tract is painful, sexual intercourse will, of course, be less enjoyable. For the partner who experiences this symptom, sexual relations may be merely a bit irritating or altogether too painful to endure. If one or both partners suffer anxiety over infertility, then sexual relations may also be less pleasurable, but this is not due to any physical cause.

If a person is infertile, he or she can sense it.

Most cases of infertility are asymptomatic. In other words, there is no way the infertile individual would be able physically to sense his or her infertility. The same situation applies to an infertile couple.

One way to overcome infertility is to have frequent intercourse.

Assuming a couple has sexual intercourse the "average" number of times—twice a week (or three times one week and one time the next week)—then a pregnancy should occur within a year. If not, then the couple is most likely suffering from an infertility problem or combination of problems, and such a problem or combination of problems is not likely to be overcome by having sexual intercourse more frequently. For possible exceptions, see below.

Carefully timing sexual intercourse to occur during the right time of the month is crucial to overcoming infertility.

Again, if a couple has sexual intercourse roughly two times a week and no specific infertility problems are involved, then coordinating sexual activity precisely with the optimum time in the female partner's monthly menstrual cycle doesn't really boost the chances of conceiving. If they're having sexual relations only twice a month, then it does make sense to time intercourse to coincide with the female partner's optimum days for conception each month.

Another situation in which timing may matter is when age is a factor—that is, when the female partner is over thirty-six. A couple perceiving a biological deadline may not want to wait as long as a year for a conception to occur. Instead, they may attempt to maximize their chances each month by timing sexual intercourse to occur on the best days. In cases where several factors come into play—for example, a low sperm count, a female partner over thirty-six, and a history of bacterial infections in either partner—then timing can make a critical difference.

Infertility can be inherited.

Infertility per se cannot be inherited, except in extremely rare cases involving structural or hormonal problems that are genetic in nature. In these cases, the problems are almost always manifestly apparent to the person who has them.

Unlike many of my colleagues, however, I do believe there is one respect in which this myth is not far from the truth. My experience with numerous patients has convinced me that harmful bacteria can be transmitted during the birthing process from a mother's reproductive system to her child's reproductive system. And abnormalities in a pregnancy (which will be clarified later) can make the offspring even more vulnerable to contamination in his or her genital tract. But this is a matter to be explored in the next chapter, where I discuss how I diagnose and treat specific cases in my practice.

Chapter 3

....

How Antibiotic Therapy Works to Ensure Fertility

Typically, when people go to a fertility specialist, they're prepared to be patients in the most literal sense of the term. They assume their task will be to wait patiently in fear, hope, and bewilderment while the specialist performs inscrutable tests on them and, ultimately, deciphers what's wrong with their reproductive system. When people come to me, their role is not a passive one at all. Instead, they join me as active partners in a detective case.

Much of the territory I want my patients to explore is predictable, given their reason for consulting me. Therefore, I can set them on the trail even before we meet. I've designed a detailed questionnaire to elicit any medical or family history relevant to a couple's current status of infertility, and I ask that the questionnaire be completed ahead of time so we can review it together during the first appointment.

The most important group of questions—for both the man and the woman—concerns previous marriages and/or relationships. I ask them to establish the order and extent of their individual sexual experiences with different partners and the kinds of birth control they practiced prior to their own sexual union.

In the woman's case, I am particularly interested in learning about any previous infectious events related to her genital tract,

39

such as vaginitis, cervicitis, PID, abdominal pain, or STD. I want to know whether she ever perceived any changes in her menstrual period—for example, she may have observed a difference in the color, pattern, or quantity of the menstrual flow, or there might have been a delay in the onset of a period, which could be interpreted as a short-lived pregnancy. I also ask her about obstetric events or premenstrual symptoms during any previous relationships. Once this past history has been covered, the woman is directed to provide similar information regarding her current relationship.

In the man's case, I am likewise interested in both the past and the recent health status of his genital tract. The questions posed to him cover the full range of male-related problems—from relatively common events, such as changes in the nature of the ejaculation, a burning sensation when urinating, urethral discharge, prostatitis, epididymitis, or testicular infection, to less common and more potentially serious conditions, such as undescended testicles, hydrocele, varicocele, or venereal disease.

Finally, the questionnaire bids the man and the woman to focus on the specific time period during which they've been trying without success to achieve a pregnancy together. They are asked more specific questions about any methods they may have used in their marriage to avoid a pregnancy as well as about their sexual practices, any previously performed infertility tests, and any medications or procedures they've tried in an effort to reverse or overcome their infertility.

Among all these latter questions, I am especially interested in knowing the length of time the man and the woman have been attempting to have a baby. Speaking strictly as a physician, I've observed that if an infectious cause does lie behind a couple's infertility, then the longer they've tried to conceive, the more extensive the infection-related damage is likely to be in the woman's reproductive tract. Speaking as a human being, I've learned from my patients that a lengthy, frustrating trial for pregnancy can destroy the spontaneous desire for intercourse and leave in its place a preplanned performance schedule mechanically timed to coordinate with ovulation. With this unfortunate side effect in mind, I rely a great deal on tact and humor to make our doctor-patient collaboration and, I hope, their sexual response to each other during this time as pleasant and casual as possible.

My patients may be uncomfortable or embarrassed about answering the questions I've mentioned so far, and they may not understand what, specifically, can be learned from individual answers, but at least the questions themselves seem relevant to their goal. They realize we need to discuss such sexual matters openly, and so my tact-and-humor formula usually works right away to make this discussion easier.

Other questions take my patients completely by surprise. For example, I may ask a male or female patient:

- Are you an only child? A first, second, or third child? A last child?

- Were you born prematurely? Were you born by cesarean section? How long was your mother in labor?

- Were you often sick as a child? Did you have frequent bouts with tonsillitis? Enlarged adenoids? Recurring ear infections?

- Where did your mother and father come from? Where did your grandparents come from?

• What is the reproductive history of your siblings?

I might ask a woman who has already borne a child whether she experienced a noticeable personality change after the delivery. I might ask a man who has fathered a child in a previous relationship whether his former partner exhibited a noticeable personality change after the delivery or whether the relationship started to suffer seriously a few months following the birth of a particular child. What could the answers to these questions possibly have to do with the patient's or couple's infertility?

In this chapter, I'll examine the reasons behind all these questions—both the predictable and the unexpected—by reviewing actual cases from my practice. I'll consider how and why individuals become involved in my antibiotic treatment program, what they experience as a result of that program, and why it makes sense as a first-step strategy for preventing and reversing infertility.

·········· LYNN: A FRESH START ··········

No matter how paramount the problem of infertility may be in their lives, most people won't discuss it in a social setting—unless they find themselves in the company of a fertility specialist. When Lynn and I first met informally in 1980, she was emboldened by years of frustration to share with me her disastrous reproductive history. It was a history she assumed was behind her, for she had ceased to menstruate the year before, at age thirty-seven, and three different specialists had told her she had suffered ovarian failure. In short, she considered herself a victim of premature menopause.

Lynn's health troubles began in 1969, when she married Richard. Prior to the marriage, Richard had been bothered by frequent episodes of nonspecific urethritis, a common inflammation of the urinary tract that, in hindsight, was probably not treated adequately. After the marriage, Lynn also began to have similar problems: lower-urinary-tract infections and vaginal irritations. She immediately became pregnant but lost the baby after four months due to a premature rupture of membranes. No fertility workup was performed; her doctor simply urged the couple to try again. In 1970, they conceived once more, but Lynn miscarried within a few weeks.

Following the failure of her second pregnancy, Lynn had her first fertility workup, which resulted in a rather broad diagnosis of luteal-phase defect—that is, a delayed development of the uterine lining. She was given progesterone, a typical medication for this condition, and was told her chances of bearing a child full term would subsequently be much better.

The strategy appeared to work: in 1972, after an eight-month pregnancy, Lynn gave premature birth to a boy. Recalling this pregnancy for me, she mentioned that her baby was conceived while she was on a short course of tetracycline for a skin problem. She remembered going to Florida shortly afterward and being forced to discontinue the tetracycline because it made her skin too sensitive to the sun. This seemingly insignificant detail stuck in my mind.

In the hospital, during her recuperation from the delivery, Lynn developed a serious infection in her uterus (endometritis). She was treated with antibiotics (ampicillin and cephalothin) and then sent home with the baby. Right after her next period, she became pregnant again. However, since neither Richard nor Lynn wanted a second child so soon, Lynn had an induced abortion.

A year later, Richard and Lynn conceived another child but lost it at fifteen weeks. Fertility specialists attributed this particular miscarriage to an incompetent cervix and advised her to get a stitch in her cervix to improve her chances of holding a fetus full term. She chose not to get the stitch. "There was no guarantee it would do any good," she explained. "Plus it would mean having to remain in bed for most of the pregnancy, which I didn't think I could manage." Instead, she opted for a heavy regimen of fertility drugs, including clomiphene and progesterone.

Over the next four years, from 1975 through 1979, Lynn had five more miscarriages. The last two pregnancies (her tenth and eleventh) were so short in duration that they could be detected only by biochemical analysis. At this point, her doctor warned her she was failing to ovulate and her menstruation was shrinking away. He prescribed Pergonal, one of the most potent fertility drugs available. Four months before we met, she had stopped taking Pergonal. She had not had a period—or sexual intercourse with her husband—since then.

Aside from all the emotional and physical pain Lynn had suffered throughout the previous ten years, something else profoundly disturbed me about her story. I couldn't reconcile its various elements: the rationale behind individual diagnoses, the sequence of diagnoses, the repeated occurrences of infection in her reproductive system, the timing of her one successful pregnancy, and the ultimate conclusion that she had irretrievably lost her reproductive powers. I finally said to her, "Why don't we look into this matter a little further?" Weary though she and her husband were of tests and treatments, they responded positively to my suggestion.

The first thing I did was perform culture studies for each partner: two apiece to ensure accuracy. Both times, Richard's semen and a biopsy from Lynn's uterine lining tested positive for chlamydia. This discovery implied it was indeed highly possible, as I'd suspected, that Lynn's reproductive difficulties were tied directly to bacterial infection.

At my recommendation, Lynn came into the hospital for a laparoscopy (a visualization of her ovaries via a telescope-like instrument); and what we learned completely contradicted the grim diagnosis of ovarian failure that had so depressed her. In fact, she had plenty of eggs—they just weren't being released from the ovary as they should be.

In June of 1981, I prescribed a broad-spectrum antibiotic drug program for Lynn and for Richard. Lynn received 100 milligrams of doxycycline twice a day for six days intravenously in the hospital followed by three weeks of the same dosage orally as an outpatient. Richard took 100 milligrams of doxycycline orally twice a day over the same time period. Meanwhile, I advised them to continue abstaining from intercourse until we had clear evidence their individual bacterial infections were completely eradicated.

Right after the treatment ended, an ecstatic Lynn phoned me to say she had resumed menstruating. An endometrial biopsy following this announcement showed her uterine lining was in good condition, possessing what is known in medical terms as perfect phase.

Enormously heartened by Lynn's progress, I said to her, "OK, go home and start having sexual intercourse with your husband." It took a few weeks before they were able to overcome two years of mutual avoidance, but in October of 1981, Lynn conceived again. To everyone's joy, after an uneventful, nine-month pregnancy, she gave birth to a healthy girl.

Looking back over the history of this case, I interpret Lynn's and Richard's reproductive problems as follows. Because Lynn had never experienced any genital-tract problems prior to her marriage and because her husband had, I reasoned that Lynn's postnuptial history of cystitis, vaginitis, and infection of the uterine lining and ovaries came from exposure to Richard's seminal fluid. Most likely, chlamydia entered Richard's seminal fluid during the time of his premarriage genital-tract infections and was never completely eliminated by the medication administered for those infections. The subsequent infection of his wife was an ascending one; that is, it began in the lowest part of her genital tract and progressed to higher and higher structures without obstructing the fallopian tubes.

The fertility workup conducted by the first specialist Lynn consulted yielded a diagnosis of a deficient uterine lining with perfectly maintained ovarian function and normal hormonal levels. Fertility workups later in her history pointed to luteal-phase defect plus a deficient hormonal supply from the ovaries, indicating that the ovaries, at this point, were now malfunctioning. Reviewing the histological slide I prepared from her specimen at the time of the laparoscopy, I saw clear evidence of bacterial infection, and ultimately, I had no doubt that her failing ovaries were being suppressed by chlamydia.

I was now able to envision mentally how a spreading bacterial infection had led to Lynn's series of miscarriages. I propose that her one pregnancy resulting in a live child, her son, was facilitated by the tetracycline she was taking when the child was conceived. In addition to clearing her skin condition, it also worked—without anyone's knowledge at the time—to suppress the chlamydia in her reproductive system, rendering her more capable of bearing a child. I further propose that the tetracycline treatment was not extensive enough to ensure a trouble-free pregnancy, and so she delivered prematurely. Whether or not the young child's chronic episodes of asthma, bronchitis, ear infection, and tonsillitis were due to intrauterine exposure to microbes is only hypothetical, but from my point of view, it could be of significant relevance.

Lynn's health history displays the whole spectrum of ways bacterial infection can spread through the female genital tract and interfere with every single step in the reproductive process. In fact, this one case is so impressive that it single-handedly triggered my interest in studying habitual aborters and the relationships between ongoing bacterial infections and simultaneously deteriorating fertility. But the fascinating scope of Lynn's case doesn't stop there. Her history also reveals a potentially strong link between bacterial infection and PMS.

Following the restoration of her normal menstrual cycle, Lynn reported that several troublesome premenstrual problems she had experienced during most of her married life had now changed for the better or had completely disappeared. Specifically, she no longer suffered so severely from breast tenderness, bloating, depression, or hostility, and she was much more enthusiastic about sexual intercourse. Analyzing her premenstrual symptoms closely, I found them to be the same symptoms that many of my own patients and medical literature in general associate with PMS. Five years passed before I could launch my first organized study into the effects of antibiotics on certain cases of PMS, but it was Lynn's case that prompted me to ask about PMS symptoms in every subsequent consultation. In Chapter 5, I will talk more about PMS and antibiotic therapy.

TREATING DIFFERENT TYPES OF
.... INFECTIONS ....

As far as Lynn is concerned, antibiotic therapy restored to health a reproductive system that had been compromised by a bacterial infection in the ovaries. Just as often in my practice, however, antibiotic therapy has reversed infertility caused by a bacterial infection somewhere else in a woman's reproductive system. The female genital tract is compartmentalized into a lower genital area, comprising the labia, the vagina, and the lower cervix, and an upper genital area, comprising the uterus and the fallopian tubes. Infections serious enough to cause—or foster—infertility can occur at several critical points along this tract.

Rita, a twenty-nine-year-old woman, came to me because of an ongoing vaginal irritation (vaginitis). She also suffered from a chronic infection of the Bartholin's gland, which is located just under the small labia and is supposed to lubricate the vaginal entrance. Both conditions made sexual intercourse intolerably painful and, therefore, thwarted her sexual satisfaction as well as her desire to have a baby.

The Bartholin's-gland problem presented the bigger treatment challenge. In cases like Rita's, we count heavily on antibiotic therapy to locate and destroy the precise bacterium that is causing the inflammation. Otherwise, surgery has to be considered. This involves opening up the infected gland and allowing the pus to drain from it over a period of time—a much more painful, expensive, and time-consuming procedure.

Rita was referred to me by a colleague and had already received three courses of oral antibiotics plus a month's supply of vaginal creams. Nothing seemed to help. As a first step, I conducted bacterial testing on both Rita and her husband, Jerry. The only meaningful isolate in both Rita's vaginal fluid and Jerry's seminal fluid was an anaerobe, streptococcus, which I decided to treat with Flagyl, a commonly used antibiotic. A two-week course of 500 milligrams four times daily was prescribed for both partners. As a result, Rita experienced temporary relief of her symptoms. A month later, I requested repeat culture studies. Unfortunately, the bacterium had reappeared. And even before the culture reports were available, Rita's symptoms had flared up again.

When I first met Rita, I was just beginning to try out a portable infusion pump for ambulatory treatment of PID. My purpose was to enable patients to live at home while they were on medication instead of having to remain in the hospital. The pump had a small reservoir containing a day's supply of clindamycin and gentamicin, the two most potent drugs for treating PID. It featured plastic tubing that carried the antibiotic solution to the patient's lower arm, where a venous catheter was inserted into a vein. On the whole, it was a fairly cumbersome apparatus, and during treatment courses, the catheter had to be changed several times. The drugs themselves can have dangerous side effects, so we had designed a very close monitoring system to follow the patients who were using it.

At that time, I had never heard of using intravenous treatment to alleviate the types of problems Rita and her husband had. But I was so frustrated with the stubborn perseverance of the anaerobic bacteria in both partners' reproductive system despite the oral regimens that I prescribed ten days on the intravenous pump for both of them. The results were spectacular. Rita's Bartholin's duct healed, her vaginitis disappeared, and follow-up cultures on both her vaginal fluid and Jerry's semen were negative for the anaerobe.

After resuming a normal intercourse pattern, Rita achieved pregnancy within four months. In retrospect, I can't help but be convinced that Rita's problems were due to an anaerobic bacterial contamination. Since she had been completely asymptomatic until entering marriage, I also believe that the original anaerobic infection came from Jerry's seminal fluid.

Now let's consider cervical infections. Because the cervix functions as the mechanical and immunological barrier between a woman's lower and upper genital tracts, it is especially vulnerable to bacterial infection, and any infection that takes hold there is highly likely to result in infertility. This is precisely what happened in the case of Keith and Becky, a couple in their early thirties who had tried for eight years to have a baby and had failed to conceive even once.

Before consulting me, Becky had undergone a laparoscopy and several hysterosalpingograms (X-ray examinations of the fallopian tubes). None of these procedures indicated any problem that would inhibit reproduction. There was, however, a persistent abnormal finding in her previous chartings. The postcoital test, which evaluates the survival of sperm in the cervical mucus, was repeatedly noted, by three different infertility specialists, to be poor or marginal at best. Vaginal douching with baking soda failed to improve sperm survival in her cervical mucus, and three cycles of intrauterine artificial insemination did not overcome her infertility.

The first thing I did after reviewing their individual and combined reproductive histories was to analyze Keith's semen and Becky's cervical mucus. Both showed high concentrations of mycoplasma and anaerobic bacteria—specifically, two anaerobes were shared, and Keith had one additional anaerobic bacterium.

In the spring of 1988, after a combined course of oral doxycycline did not improve the postcoital test and did not eradicate the anaerobic organisms, I put Becky and Keith on two weeks of intravenous clindamycin and gentamicin. Subsequently, I tested them again for mycoplasma and anaerobic bacteria. This time, the results were negative, and a postcoital test was excellent in all respects. In August of 1988, Becky became pregnant, and nine months later to the day I delivered a healthy boy.

My summary of Keith and Becky's case is that a chronic cervical infection with local antibody formation resulted in their infertility. Following the antibiotic therapy, we tested Becky's cervical mucus and her blood for antisperm antibodies, and they were negative. If, as in this case, only the cervix is contaminated and the immune system is not yet involved, antibiotic therapy can usually result in pregnancy within a few months. If infection is documented in both the cervix and the uterine lining, however, especially with antisperm antibodies already detected, patients may have to wait six to ten months after antibiotic therapy before a pregnancy can be expected. In my opinion, this extended time is necessary for the complete cessation of antibody production.

THE ISSUE OF VERTICAL
.... TRANSMISSION ....

In the cases I've reviewed so far, information provided by my patients relating directly to their sexual and reproductive history enabled me to suspect what culture studies confirmed— that bacteria had been continuously exchanged between one partner and another during intercourse and had eventually created an infection virulent enough to cause infertility. Often in such cases, I can deduce from the initial interview precisely how the bacteria spread.

For example, if a woman first develops vaginal irritation after marrying a man who had recurrent bouts with STDs during his bachelor days, it's logical for me to posit that she picked up infectious agents from her husband. If a woman taking birth control pills tells me that she always avoids sexual intercourse during menstruation, then I can assume with reasonable surety that any infection she may have contracted while taking the pills has not spread above her cervix. If an infertile woman has previously borne a child, I know one strong possibility is that bacterial infection, transmitted to the woman at the time of conception, ascended through her reproductive system and intensified.

But how do I explain the apparent presence of bacterial infection in the reproductive tract of a woman who by every indication has no history of sexual contact or reproduction at all? The only explanation lies in vertical transmission, the passage of bacteria from parent to child during fetal development and/or the birthing process itself.

52

The scientific community unanimously agrees that bacteria can be transmitted to the ear canal, nasal passages, oral cavities, and gastrointestinal tract by way of the newborn's swallowing the genital-tract fluid of the mother. Speculation that the baby's genital tract is another body orifice that can be colonized by the mother's bacteria is compelling but far more complicated to verify. Assuming, as I do, that this transmission does indeed occur, then it is perhaps the most mysterious aspect of bacterial infection in the reproductive system, and the effort to shed some light on that mystery accounts for the more surprising questions I ask my patients.

Irene was a virgin. Her mother brought her to me because she had been suffering erratic menstrual periods, with profuse bleeding and unusually long bleeding times, since she was sixteen—about a year and a half after menarche. I was as positive as I could be from appearances, examination results, and interview material that she had led a very wholesome and sheltered life and, at the age of eighteen, had yet to experience physical intimacy with a man. When I accepted her as a patient, the fact that there were situations where bacteria could be transmitted vertically was just beginning to be acknowledged. Faced with the enigma of Irene's symptoms, I said to myself, Let me begin by investigating her family history.

Irene, it turns out, was an only child. Her mother's menstrual periods had ceased at the relatively young age of thirty-seven, an event that was written off as premature ovarian failure and menopause. Irene's father had been the victim of episodic prostatitis for most of his life. I conjectured that the source of both parents' health problems was bacterial infection. Specifically, I theorized that the bacteria had been passed from the father to the mother and had ascended to the mother's upper genital tract during the course of her pregnancy with Irene, rendering her infertile thereafter.

As for Irene herself, I suspected even before testing her that her menstrual troubles were due to an infection resulting from prenatal exposure to her mother's bacteria. Sure enough, the bacteria culture revealed five different anaerobic bacteria in her vaginal tract. I prescribed a ten-week program of oral antibiotics: three weeks of Vibra-Tabs, followed by three weeks of erythromycin, followed by two weeks of Flagyl and another course of erythromycin. Within one month after completing the last antibiotic course, her specific menstrual irregularity disappeared, and she resumed a normal menstrual pattern.

While taking Irene's history during our initial consultation, I learned that a previous specialist had recommended birth control pills to alleviate her perplexing menstrual difficulties. She followed this advice but found the pills emotionally upsetting. So did her mother, a conservative woman and protective parent who kept complaining to the specialist, "My daughter's a virgin. Why in heaven's name should she be put on birth control pills?" Fortunately, Irene stopped taking the pills after a few months (as a substitute, her specialist prescribed a dilation and curettage—D and C—to alleviate cramps and Danocrine for possible endometriosis). Had she remained on the pills, her condition would have been superficially indiscernible, making her feel her troubles had been eliminated while, in reality, the bacteria present in her genital tract would have continued to proliferate.

This case has an especially rewarding coda. Two years after I treated Irene's infection, she was astute enough to return to my laboratory with her fiancé, Tom, so that he, too, could be checked for possible bacterial contamination. Tom's test revealed no such problem. After their marriage, they conceived during the first month they stopped using condoms. One day shy of the due date, Irene gave birth to a healthy girl. A chain of infection passing from parent to child—for who knows how many generations—is now broken.

As convincing an example of vertical transmission as Irene's case may be, it was impossible to prove she actually picked up infectious bacteria from her mother. I couldn't insist that her parents come in for bacteria cultures. At any rate, her mother had had a hysterectomy many years before, so obtaining the culture I needed from her would have been impossible, and her father's strict religious beliefs prevented him from discussing his daughter's situation, much less becoming actively involved in it.

Even assuming Irene's mother had not had a hysterectomy, and both parents had volunteered to be tested, and the resulting cultures had contained the same kinds of anaerobic bacteria, it's purely a matter of speculation that the parents' bacteria found their way into the child's reproductive system. Current technology does not enable us to trace a literal parent-child link between one group of bacteria and another or to observe bacteria in the process of moving from mother to child before or during birth. Nevertheless, the circumstantial evidence supporting vertical transmission is overwhelming.

As it happens, my very first private patient in the United States wound up contributing to that body of evidence. Barbara was already pregnant when I took over her case in the summer of 1976—I was covering for a colleague of mine on an extended vacation. At six and a half months' gestation,

Barbara was hospitalized with premature labor. We couldn't halt her labor with the methods available to us then (intravenous alcohol, sedation, and bed rest), so we soon were forced to deliver a tiny female child, Alice, who spent the next three weeks in the hospital's intensive-care unit before going home.

Alice was destined to be an only child. Later, Barbara consulted me about chronic vaginal irritation dating from the time Alice was born. I cultured Barbara and discovered chlamydia in her vagina. In 1988, Alice herself, now twelve years old, came to my laboratory. She had just begun menstruating, and her vaginal discharge was disturbingly copious and odd smelling. Although she was a virgin, she, too, tested positive for chlamydia.

In my opinion, the only sensible explanation for Alice's infection is that she had harbored chlamydia in her reproductive system since contracting it from her mother, most likely in the womb itself during the turbulence attending her mother's premature labor. Twelve years later, the onset of Alice's sexual maturity triggered changes in her vaginal milieu that were favorable to the chlamydia bacteria and caused them to flourish to the extent that they gave her the localized symptoms I've already mentioned.

In the interest of scientific accuracy, I must repeat that vertical transmission of bacteria from the genital tract of the mother to the genital tract of the child is technically a theory, not an established fact. Patients concerned about their individual fertility problems are understandably, if lamentably, reluctant to involve family members in such a highly sensitive area of their lives. Within the limits of my own practice, which is large and cosmopolitan, I have been able to obtain matching cultures from only six mother–virgin-daughter pairs and only one complete family unit: a father, a mother, and their virgin daughter, who all tested positive for chlamydia. I consider myself lucky to have achieved this much progress.

Yet, as a scientist, I must also admit I support the vertical-transmission hypothesis because it reconciles so many diverse phenomena that crop up in the histories of infertile people. Hundreds of successful diagnoses and treatments have stemmed from my belief in this hypothesis, and that fact alone explains why I initially ask my patients the more surprising questions cited at the beginning of this chapter—questions having to do with the reproductive health history of the patients' parents and siblings and the circumstances surrounding the patients' birth.

Let's suppose, for example, a woman develops amnionitis in the sixth month of her pregnancy. In other words, the amniotic fluid that surrounds the baby and protects the baby from infection is itself contaminated with bacteria. The baby already has some kind of immune system working, the specific organs being the bronchial tree, the nasal pharynx, the lymphatic tissues, the ear canal, the prostate in a male, and the cervix in a female. All of these organs are suddenly at risk for infection.

Possibly the mother we are discussing will go into early labor at this point. If so, chances are good she will be given paralyzing agents to prolong her pregnancy, which may leave the baby soaking in the infected fluid for weeks or even months to come. Whatever the labor and delivery situation, the baby may be born with any number of immunological maladies—manifest or not—that could indicate bacterial infection in the reproductive system as well: chronic coughing, bronchitis, postnasal drip, allergies, oversized tonsils or adenoids, an enlarged prostate, an irritated cervix.

If the baby is fortunate enough to be saved from bacterial infection by way of the amniotic fluid, he or she is subject to infectious exposure from the second the membrane ruptures. If a cesarean section is performed on the mother, the risk of the baby becoming infected during the birth process is very low. In a vaginal delivery, the risk of infection is, in my estimation, very high—and increases the longer the labor lasts.

So we see why I ask my patients how long their mother was in labor and whether there were any complications surrounding their birth. After conducting some family research of her own, one patient, Andrea, responded, "My mother went into labor, then stopped, then was stimulated with Pitocin. The membrane at this stage had already broken. After another hour, she was told to go to sleep for the night. I wasn't born until late the following day." Andrea herself had been plagued with tonsillitis, colic, and ear infections as a child and had developed vaginitis during puberty. When I cultured her, I found a high level of mycoplasma.

Taking all this data into account, I felt the final picture strongly suggested that Andrea was infected with mycoplasma from her mother, whose pregnancy with Andrea may have been complicated by mycoplasmal infection. By the time Andrea was finally ready to have a child of her own, the mycoplasma inside her reproductive system had long since caused an infection that prevented her from conceiving. The antibiotic therapy I prescribed wiped out the mycoplasma, the infection disappeared, and she became pregnant shortly afterward.

If my patient or either of my patient's parents (or my patient's partner or either of his or her parents) is an only child, then I know it's possible I'm dealing with a family history of secondary infertility due to bacterial infection. I'm also alert to the possibility of vertical transmission if I learn my patient's siblings (or his or her partner's siblings) have had childless or one-child marriages. But what could I hope to gain from a patient's answer to the question, "Where are your parents from?" or "What is your ancestry?"

Essentially, I'm trying to investigate the origin of my patient's physical being as thoroughly as I can, so I can be all the more confident about my diagnosis of his or her reproductive health problem and about the potential efficacy of solving that problem with broad-spectrum antibiotic treatment. Perhaps one or both of my patient's parents were from an extremely inbred community or cultural group, in which case the chance of vertical transmission of bacteria or the chance of vertical transmission of a genetic condition predisposing the recipient to bacterial infection is much greater.

It is my impression, based on my own experience and research into the matter, that patients who can trace their descent to tropical, tribal areas, like the South Pacific or Africa, are far more likely to be heavily laden with vertically transmitted bacteria in general than patients whose families come from temperate, nontribal areas. I also believe (again, based on my own experience and research) that descendants of people who were incarcerated in concentration camps fall into a more contaminated category.

This entire line of inquiry is clearly controversial. It must be pursued however—with extra sensitivity and scrupulosity, to be sure—if we are to accept the possibility that infectious bacteria can be transmitted vertically to the child's reproductive tract.

THE ISSUE OF "PERSONALITY .... CHANGE" ....

Not all of the questions that surprise my patients are aimed at tracing vertical transmission. Some are concerned with establishing horizontal (or sexual) transmission, which can reveal itself in many unsuspected ways. The questions of this type that raise the most eyebrows among my patients deal with postpregnancy personality changes.

When I ask a female patient who has previously given birth whether she noticed any change in her personality after the delivery, I am trying to decipher whether she might have begun experiencing PMS at that time. If she admits having noticed a personality change and the change corresponds to the type of troublesome emotional patterns commonly associated with PMS, then I can hypothesize that her pregnancy spurred the development of a serious bacterial infection that caused her to develop PMS—and, perhaps, secondary infertility as well.

When I ask a male patient whether he witnessed any change in his partner's personality, or in that of any prior partner after she gave birth, I am attempting to find out whether she might have developed PMS at that time, which could indicate that the two of them exchanged infectious bacteria during the course of their sexual relationship. I usually pose this question without explaining in advance why I'm asking it, so I don't prejudice the response. As a result of this strategy and of the professional knowledge that lies behind my questioning, I can sometimes appear to be psychic.

Recently, I was conducting an initial interview with a patient, Paul, who said he had previously been involved in a four-year marriage that produced one male child before ending in divorce. As soon as I heard this, I said to him, "Am I correct in assuming your first wife went into a severe depression after delivering your son?" He was clearly taken aback. "How did you know that?" he asked. I told him it was just a guess. Then I went on to inquire, "Is it fair to say that about six months later, you were fighting all the time, and your marriage was going on the rocks?" Speechless, he nodded.

Ultimately, I collected enough data from my interview with Paul to justify a preliminary conclusion that his ex-wife had developed PMS after her pregnancy—and, therefore, possibly harbored a bacterial infection in her reproductive system. Then Paul mentioned that his son from that marriage is a "problem child," subject to all sorts of infectious diseases and the ill-tempered behavior that often goes with them. This additional information only corroborated my suspicion that bacteria were transmitted through the family. I wasn't surprised in the least when I subsequently discovered high levels of chlamydia in Paul's semen.

Only in recent years has PMS been acknowledged as a legitimate physical illness with potentially devastating emotional consequences. Given the lack of popular understanding concerning PMS, it's little wonder so many cases of it are never recognized as such by their victims or their mates. The consequences of such ignorance can be enormous, for identifying PMS is frequently an important step toward identifying even more serious conditions, including infertility. I'll return to the subject of PMS in Chapter 5, where I'll also examine other reproductive health problems short of infertility that can be successfully managed with high-powered antibiotic treatment.

ANTIBIOTIC TREATMENT TO RESTORE FERTILITY: .... WHAT TO EXPECT ....

By discussing the questions—common and uncommon—I ask my patients, I hope that I have provided some insight into the range of issues that need to be examined before I can determine (a) the most probable cause of a patient's infertility and (b) the specific antibiotic therapy most likely to alleviate or eliminate that cause. Now it's time to consider what my patients want to know about antibiotic treatment programs in general.

Here are the questions I most often encounter from my patients or prospective patients, accompanied by my responses:

What symptoms may indicate I have a bacterial infection in my genital tract?

The most important point to remember concerning this issue is that a bacterial infection harmful enough to interfere with fertility does not necessarily announce itself in ways you can feel or observe. In my experience, vertically transmitted bacterial flora in particular is scarcely ever symptomatic. Therefore, the procedure I recommend is to begin your self-examination by considering whether you might be in a high-risk category for congenital reasons.

Here are some questions to ask yourself (and, perhaps, members of your family or a family physician):

1. Am I an only child? Why?

2. Were there miscarriages before and/or after my birth?

3. Was I born prematurely?

4. Did my mother have any unusually severe infection around the time I was born?

5. Did my mother try to get pregnant for a long time before I was born? Were my parents trying to overcome any infections during this period?

If a bacterium transmitted at birth remains in the genital tract of the adolescent, usually that person's very first sexual partner will pick it up and develop symptoms from it. In a male partner, the most common symptom of such a sexually transmitted infection is a burning sensation when urinating or soreness in the urinary tract and, later, prostatitis. A female partner might develop what is commonly labeled a yeast infection (vaginitis).

If you are a woman and you experienced a vaginal infection or repeated episodes of cystitis around puberty—and prior to any history of sexual intercourse—then this may be a symptomatic warning sign of vertically transmitted bacterial infection. Whatever your age now, you should definitely arrange to be cultured for bacteria.

If you are a DES-exposed child, I also recommend being tested for the presence of infectious agents in your genital tract. The drug known as DES (diethylstilbestrol, a synthetic estrogen) was widely administered during the 1950s to pregnant women who had a history of miscarrying. The drug did, indeed, work to prevent miscarriage, but tragically for the individuals it helped to bring into the world, it caused a high rate of infertility, which fertility specialists often attribute to anatomical malformations in the reproductive system.

The reason I advise bacteria testing for DES-exposed children is not that I suspect any possible adverse effect of the DES itself. I believe the infertility problem many of them experience results from the same condition for which the DES was given to their mothers—a bacterial infection causing a tendency to miscarry. The DES ingested by the mother maintained the child artificially inside an infected uterus until birth, a situation that, in my opinion, would almost certainly have resulted in heavy bacterial contamination of the child by way of vertical transmission. I have treated numerous DES-exposed women whose spontaneous abortions had been written off by previous specialists as the effects of a DES-related malformed uterus (the so-called T-shaped uterus) or an incompetent cervix. In every single case to date, a strong course of antibiotic therapy has yielded a normal pregnancy.

After identifying all factors that might suggest vertical transmission of bacterial infection, look for indicators of possible sexual transmission. Consider your history of sexual partners and sexual activities in conjunction with any unusual physical symptoms you may have experienced in the genital or pelvic area.

For men, episodes of urethritis, prostatitis, or gonorrhea are

64

especially suspect for asymptomatic bacterial infection. For women, the most telling indicators are chronically recurring vaginitis (yeast infection) or repeated flare-ups of PID. Any deviation from "normal" menstruation is also suspicious: for example, a time when the menstrual flow suddenly became lighter, heavier, or more odorous or when the cycle itself became irregular or studded with midcycle bleeding. Menstruation that turns into brown staining almost always suggests endometritis or ovarian infection. Other functional problems that can be associated with bacterial infection are ovarian-cyst formation, a rapidly developing luteal-phase defect, or the skipping of ovulation altogether (anovulatory cycles).

Women also need to review their history of birth control. IUD users, past or present, are in a high-risk category for bacterial infection. Women who use barrier-type birth control, such as condoms or diaphragms, should be concerned if any sudden change in pelvic function occurs after they discontinue use. Ideally, a woman experiencing such a symptom should immediately refrain from sexual intercourse and go for testing.

In cases of secondary infertility, the course of the first pregnancy frequently provides clues that mandate the search for bacteria. In general, the longer it took to conceive the child, with all fertility parameters being normal, the higher the chance the secondary infertility is bacteria-related. Other abnormalities surrounding a first pregnancy that may indicate bacterial infection are unusual bleeding, prematurity, postdatism, an incompetent cervix, intrauterine growth retardation of the fetus, an exceptionally long labor without an oversized fetus, a cesarean section performed for reasons besides size differentials, and postpartum infections of the mother or the newborn.

So far, we've been considering mild bacterial infections. Severe bacterial infections in the female genital tract invariably cause clinically discernible symptoms, including pain, fever, localized tenderness, an elevated sedimentation rate, a high white-cell count in the blood, and/or copious vaginal discharge. A more subtle, but still manifest symptom is an emotional and, sometimes, physical disturbance during the weeks preceding a period, which could betoken PMS. (See Chapter 5 for a more specific discussion of PMS symptoms.)

Assuming I don't notice any specific symptoms and I can't account for possible bacterial infection by reviewing my family or sexual history, when should I consider being checked for bacterial infection in my genital tract?

The ideal situation is for a man or woman to be cultured shortly after puberty and definitely before sexual intercourse begins. Of course, this scenario requires parents who are informed about the possible causes and effects of bacterial infection. Whether or not you had this experience, your approach to testing should be preventive rather than strictly curative.

I recommend yearly examination of seminal fluid for sexually active men and yearly examination of vaginal and cervical cultures for sexually active women. In the woman's case, these tests could be administered as additions to the annual checkup now recommended by the American College of Obstetricians and Gynecologists.

Following satisfactory results, it would be wise to determine the genital-tract flora of every new partner before engaging in sexual intercourse. If sexual intercourse causes local irritation or if you and your partner intend to have a child together, then in my opinion, a bacterial study is mandatory—the sooner, the better.

Is antibiotic therapy ever useful for just one person as opposed to a couple?

Assuming the individual being treated is—or may become—sexually active, my answer is unequivocally *no*.

Is every fertility specialist willing to consider—and prepared to offer—antibiotic therapy as a possible treatment for reversing infertility?

This is a question you must pose to individual specialists. Each doctor offers his or her own repertoire of treatments, according to the areas in which he or she feels the most knowledgeable and the most skilled. My broad-spectrum antibiotic therapy is relatively new in the field, and so not every fertility specialist has yet given it a sufficient amount of consideration or incorporated it into his or her practice. I am very gratified to see, however, the high rate at which more and more specialists are turning to broad-spectrum antibiotic therapy as a first step in restoring fertility.

About how much does antibiotic therapy cost?

Since there are no pretest guarantees regarding how much antibiotic therapy may cost you, let's take the most extreme case. Assuming your antibiotic testing calls for intravenous treatment (instead of no treatment at all or orally administered treatment) as well as a full complement of pre- and post-therapy culture studies, the final cost could be as high as three thousand dollars per person.

The majority of cases by far do not cost nearly as much. But even the top possible cost of three thousand dollars is a small price to pay if you take into account that antibiotic therapy could prevent years of frustration, the total loss of spontaneous

67

reproduction, the need for much more expensive therapies (like fertility-drug treatments or in vitro fertilization), the delivery of a premature infant, and the cost of caring for a premature or seriously infected infant in a high-risk nursery.

About how long does it take to make a diagnosis? To complete the antibiotic treatment itself? When can I resume having intercourse?

If we reasonably assume from our first look at a culture that bacterial infection may be a contributing cause of infertility, the final testing for specific organisms will take about a month. The prescribed antibiotic therapy, if given orally (which is most often the case), will take from six to eight weeks. The post-therapy testing will take another month, and only thereafter do I advise resuming unprotected intercourse—that is, intercourse without a condom.

I must add that it can take up to ten months before a pregnancy is realized. While a bacterial infection is rife in a woman's reproductive system it causes certain immunological changes, and such changes always take time to reverse themselves.

Can I pursue other types of testing or treatment for infertility while I am undergoing antibiotic therapy?

Generally, I advise my patients not to pursue other tests or treatments while they are undergoing antibiotic therapy. In the first place, other tests or treatments might neutralize or work against antibiotic therapy or render the results of the therapy inconclusive. Some tests or treatments involving invasive instruments might even spread an existing bacterial infection farther into the reproductive system. In the second place, antibiotic therapy—in my experience—has a good chance of working all by itself to restore fertility, in which case other tests and treatments are unnecessary.

In addition to refraining from unprotected sexual intercourse during antibiotic therapy, should I avoid any other activities, circumstances, or substances?

I recommend a regular diet with minimal alcohol intake. Certain tetracycline drugs that may be used in antibiotic therapy make patients sensitive to sun exposure, and because most antibiotics make the user more prone to fatigue than usual, one should minimize strenuous exercise.

Are there any negative side effects or aftereffects with antibiotic therapy?

Most of the antibiotics used in this kind of therapy can cause minor, short-term episodes of nausea, dizziness, and fatigue. Among all the antibiotics that can be used, very few produce any major side effects. In some gastrointestinal tracts, certain antibiotics may induce serious diarrhea, which ceases as soon as the patient is taken off the offending antibiotic.

Extremely high concentrations of antibiotics have the potential of damaging the kidneys or nerve endings in the ear, but this kind of dangerous situation is avoided entirely if antibiotic levels in the bloodstream are carefully monitored. This precaution always accompanies antibiotic therapy as I apply it.

Assuming both my partner and I are cleared of any bacterial infection and remain faithful to each other, might there ever be a need to repeat antibiotic therapy?

If a monogamous relationship exists and if you do not practice anal intercourse, manipulation of the genital canals with foreign objects, or oral intercourse, then your genital tract and that of your partner should remain functional and clean without the need for future testing. If an infectious symptom does recur under these circumstances, then it does not indicate re-infection but, rather, the incomplete treatment of the previous infection, in which case you should go back for testing.

If you are unable to achieve a pregnancy within a reasonable amount of time after antibiotic therapy and there is no other apparent cause for infertility, then I recommend culture studies be repeated after six months. If the same bacteria show up again, I advise repeating the antibiotic therapy.

Chapter 4

....

Paths to Parenthood:
Antibiotic Therapy and Its Options and Follow-ups

For patients and doctors alike, the quest to overcome infertility is a passionate one involving not only a struggle on the physical plane but also a struggle on the emotional plane. Each month without a pregnancy brings another wave of depression—as if a small death has occurred—and prompts another round of the same frustrating questions: Why wasn't the therapy effective? What can be done now? What is the prospect for success in the future? And each new step in therapy, whether it goes in the same direction as a previous step or in a different direction entirely, inspires fresh hope, which, in turn, calls for renewed commitment.

The prospect of creating a baby is so exciting that it compels both patients and their doctors to consider every means of restoring fertility, from the simplest to the most complicated. Weighing against that consideration, however, are very pressing limits in time, energy, and circumstances. Each couple brings its own combination of biological factors to an attempted pregnancy, and each couple that fails to achieve a pregnancy spontaneously develops its own set of decision-making criteria for getting help.

As I've stated before, fertility therapy is based on meticulous, systematic detective work. Individual leads may have to be followed from all possible angles, and individual problem-solving strategies may have to be tried again and again before a proper diagnosis is attained, reproductive health restored, and an actual pregnancy achieved. Many infertility patients and doctors understandably lack the patience to pursue this work for long periods of time, maybe years, against ever-di-minishing odds. This is especially true of female patients over the age of thirty-five (approximately 50 percent of all infertil-ity patients), who legitimately believe they can't spare much time for therapy.

It almost always takes several years for a situation causing infertility to develop in the reproductive system of a man or a woman. Restoring the health of that system, which is the best way to guarantee a healthy pregnancy and a healthy baby, also takes time: thinking time, acting time, and waiting time. Any responsible infertility treatment program requires a carefully constructed master plan that incorporates these time factors and determines the types of therapy to try first, second, and so on. Such a plan inevitably assumes a pyramidal shape, with the broadest range of appropriate therapies for a given patient at the bottom, and gradually narrows—in pace with diagnostic discoveries and/or trial-and-error experiences—to the "last re-sort" therapies at the top.

Antibiotic treatment, in my estimation, is the proper "first block, first tier" therapy in any pyramid plan to reverse infer-tility. It is the easiest and least expensive therapy; it has the least significant possible side effects; and if it doesn't eventu-ally reverse infertility, it definitely contributes to the safety and success of all other infertility treatments. Nevertheless, it can, in some cases, take a year and a half for antibiotic therapy to result in a pregnancy: approximately four months to clean the reproductive system and nine to fourteen months for the micromilieu in the genital tract to recover so a healthy pregnancy can take place spontaneously. At the top of the pyramid, by contrast, is the complex and expensive strategy known as in vitro fertilization.

Ideally, every pyramid plan to reverse infertility should be undertaken step by step, exploiting the full possibilities of each therapy before moving on to the next, more advanced and more risky therapy. There are certain situations, however, when patients must make wrenching judgments about whether to commit themselves to the full plan. Most in vitro programs, for example, won't accept a woman over forty years old, and so I am obliged to ask my female patients who are thirty-eight or thirty-nine, "Do you feel you can afford to stay with me until your fortieth birthday?" It's a decision only they can make, and only after they have reached an understanding of all the options available to them in a full plan for reversing infertility. If they do answer *no,* however, I still encourage them to go through microbial testing and antibiotic therapy to improve their chances for success with in vitro fertilization.

In this chapter, I'll examine how antibiotic therapy works in conjunction with—or in place of—other therapies to restore fertility. For the sake of convenience, I have divided this discussion into three sections, reflecting the three main categories of alternative therapies. In ascending order of complexity, these categories are: (a) fertility drugs, (b) surgery, and (c) assisted reproduction (which includes artificial insemination and in vitro fertilization).

.... FERTILITY DRUGS ....

Essentially, fertility drugs are used to compensate for hormonal imbalances in the male or female reproductive system. The biggest challenge facing specialists who administer drug therapy is to determine the proper drug dosage for each individual patient. If the dosage is too high, it may trigger negative side effects, such as overstimulation of the reproductive system and continued infertility.

The major drugs prescribed for both women and men are clomiphene, Pergonal, and human chorionic gonadotropin, or HCG. Other fertility drugs prescribed solely for women include progesterone supplements, Danocrine, and Parlodel. Obviously, fertility drugs work differently for men than they do for women, so let's consider each gender separately.

Women

Clomiphene When a woman's reproductive system is basically functional but needs stimulation—either she is ovulating erratically, or she is not ovulating at all—clomiphene is the drug treatment of choice. Clomiphene acts through the hypothalamus and pituitary glands to stimulate gonadotropin release, which in turn facilitates regular ovulation. Gonadotropin also facilitates the ovary's output of progesterone during the luteal phase, so the fertilized egg can remain securely implanted in the uterine lining.

Specific clomiphene treatment programs, like treatment programs for any fertility drug, vary greatly from individual to individual. A hypothetically valid treatment might be a daily oral dose of 50 milligrams for five days, beginning around the fifth day of the patient's monthly cycle, during the first several months of treatment. If no pregnancy occurs after three months, then the dose is usually increased for the following three months—a process that may continue until the dose is as high as 150 milligrams. Any time after that first unsuccessful month, the attending doctor may also decide to supplement the clomiphene dosage with HCG or a combination of Pergonal and HCG.

Clomiphene in low doses is a relatively harmless and complication-free medication, but when the dose reaches 100 or 150 milligrams per day for a five-day period, the patient often develops ovarian cysts. Therefore, many physicians recommend sonographic evaluation during each of several low-dosage months prior to initiating a renewed cycle with a higher dose. If the monthly sonogram shows that a patient's ovaries are free of cysts, then her clomiphene dose for the following month can be increased.

A postcoital mucus examination should also be performed for all clomiphene users during the first month and any subsequent month when the dose is increased. Clomiphene tends to have a negative effect on the cervical mucus, and thus, several months of frustration can be avoided if a poor postcoital test is documented at the very beginning and steps are taken to avert future complications.

To document the effectiveness of clomiphene on a patient's reproductive system, another very useful test is the endometrial biopsy, which the fertility specialist should perform during the second part of the patient's cycle in order to establish whether

77

the stimulation is adequate. If a favorable luteal phase is indicated by the biopsy, then there is no need to increase the patient's clomiphene dose or administer a more powerful medication.

Pergonal. A much stronger drug that works directly on the ovaries in place of the system's naturally generated hormones is Pergonal. It encourages the production of multiple eggs—an event known as superovulation—thus increasing the odds of both fertilization and a multiple pregnancy (in the case of multiple pregnancy, the chances are between 1 and 8 percent).

Pergonal is a very potent drug, and its effect on a given individual's reproductive system is highly unpredictable. Each month a patient takes Pergonal, her system's response to the drug must be closely monitored with blood tests, ultrasound scans, and mucus examinations, necessitating several visits to the fertility specialist's office.

My most common treatment regimen involving Pergonal is as follows:

1. In a given month, the patient takes 50 milligrams of clomiphene on days 2, 3, and 4 of her cycle in order to initiate ovarian stimulation.

2. Each day from day 5 to day 9 of her cycle, the patient receives 150 units of Pergonal intramuscularly.

3. During the next few days in her cycle, the patient is monitored closely with sonographic examinations. If the sonography does not show adequate ovarian stimulation by day 10, I administer Pergonal for two additional days and repeat the sonography. Pergonal administration is continued

until the sonography reveals a sufficient ovarian response, at which point I give the patient an HCG injection to facilitate release of the egg.

HCG. HCG stimulates egg maturation as well as the rupture of the egg follicle—an event that not only sends the egg on its journey to the uterus but also triggers production of progesterone, a hormone that enables the uterine lining to receive and support the egg. Most often, the patient receives an HCG injection as the final component of a clomiphene- or Pergonal-based treatment program. The moment of injection is carefully calculated so that the HCG performs its mission at the best possible time, which is approximately thirty-six hours later.

Progesterone Supplements. Progesterone in the form of pills, injections, or suppositories is often prescribed for inadequate luteal-phase function when it is feared that low natural progesterone levels may result in miscarriage.

Danocrine. Danocrine is the most common medication used to treat endometriosis, which can forestall egg development altogether. Unfortunately, being a powerful anabolic steroid, it can also cause negative side effects (including facial hair growth or muscle enlargement) in over half of the women who use it.

Parlodel. Commonly known as bromocriptine, Parlodel is used to suppress prolactin—a normal pituitary hormone that markedly elevates during pregnancy, causing engorgement of the breasts and preparation for lactation. If an excessive prolactin secretion exists prior to the onset of pregnancy, it may interfere with successful ovulation or egg implantation.

Parlodel is administered all through the monthly cycle in daily, divided doses of 2.5 milligrams. During this time, the blood prolactin level is frequently checked to make sure the desired effect is achieved.

Although I advocate giving priority to antibiotic therapy over any kind of fertility-drug therapy, I do not deny that fertility-drug therapy all by itself may enable a woman to conceive and give birth to a live baby. Nor do I deny that fertility-drug therapy is sometimes required to make this happen. I only object to the frequent practice of turning to fertility-drug therapy first, thereby seeking to override a health problem instead of trying to cure it.

Assuming, as I do, that bacterial infection causes or aggravates up to 50 percent of reproductive maladies, then it only makes sense to look for bacterial infection before going any further, especially since eradicating such an infection involves much milder medications and a much simpler treatment program. At best, antibiotic therapy alone can clear the way for a natural, safe, and comfortable pregnancy and the birth of an infant free of bacterial contamination. At the very least, antibiotic therapy increases the odds that other, subsequent treatment programs will be successful: they won't spread or intensify an already entrenched bacterial infection, their effectiveness won't be compromised or nullified by it, and they won't bring into the world a bacteria-ridden child.

Because my laboratory is a popular referral center, I have had the chance to follow the protocols of hundreds of my colleagues who deal with infertile couples. Consequently, I have been informed of several treatment regimens involving fertility drugs of which I cannot approve. There are four common situations involving clomiphene prescription that particularly bother me:

1. Many couples who consult a gynecologist after years of infertility are simply given clomiphene and sent home with the reassurance that the drug can improve their fertility.

2. Many couples are automatically given clomiphene for secondary infertility following the birth of a live baby.

3. Many couples are automatically given clomiphene after a second pregnancy ends in miscarriage, the first pregnancy having produced a live baby.

4. In cases of couples in which the woman has one malfunctioning fallopian tube, clomiphene is frequently prescribed to ensure ovulation in the ovary facing the working tube. While this increases the short-term likelihood of conception, it does not address the issue of the blocked tube.

In all four of these situations, no attempt is made by the specialist to elucidate in any detail what the cause (or causes) of the couple's previous problems may have been. In the third situation, the specialist is apparently just assuming that the lining of the uterus is too weak to maintain the pregnancy. In the fourth situation, the infectious cause of the blocked tube is ignored and no attempt is made to document whether the uterine cavity and the contralateral tube are free of harmful bacteria.

While fertility drugs are geared toward rectifying a particular problem in the genital tract and, therefore, a specific difficulty in the reproductive process, antibiotics have a pervasive effect.

A given course of antibiotic treatment eliminates harmful bacteria throughout the genital tract so the entire reproductive process can run more smoothly.

To illustrate this important distinction, let's consider reproductive health problems at different locations in the female genital tract, starting at the beginning point with a very widespread and basic problem: a vaginal milieu that is too acidic. The academic approach is to blame the acidity for killing sperm and to recommend a baking-soda douche. This relatively homespun medication will certainly make the vaginal milieu temporarily more alkaline after each application, during which time sperm entering the vagina can survive longer. My challenge to this approach is, Why not get rid of the acidity once and for all? It is quite likely bacteria are causing the acidity; so to reverse the condition permanently rather than merely to attempt overcoming it for a while, I would advise a more efficacious strategy: first, establish the presence of infectious bacteria; then, destroy those bacteria with the appropriate antibiotic regimen.

Let's move farther up the female reproductive system to a more complicated problem. Suppose a postcoital specimen of cervical mucus reveals only dead or sluggish sperm. Typically, the mucus is diagnosed as hostile, and Pergonal or estrogen is prescribed to stimulate or supplement the body's natural production of estrogen. More estrogen makes the cervical mucus more copious, diluting the concentration of any hostile agents, such as sperm antibodies or infectious bacteria. The hope is that the dilution all by itself will weaken the power of the hostile agents to harm sperm so extensively. Again, I beg to differ with this therapeutic approach. Why not take the eminently sensible precaution of checking the mucus for infectious bacteria? If the underlying problem does prove to be bacteria, it can be solved more simply and successfully with the right antibiotics.

The same argument applies to problems in the upper reproductive tract. In the uterus, luteal-phase defect may be treated—at various stages in the cycle—with clomiphene, Pergonal, progesterone supplements, and/or HCG. The basic effect of each of these drugs is to throw the uncooperative uterine lining into overdrive. By contrast, antibiotic therapy stands a good chance of eliminating the problem without risking the potentially dangerous consequences of forcing events that are not occurring naturally. Aside from tissue irritation and swelling, adverse side effects from fertility drugs might include actually jeopardizing, rather than enhancing, the system's ability to carry out a healthy pregnancy.

As for the ovaries, any of the drugs I just mentioned may be prescribed to stimulate ovarian function artificially; indeed, the problems fertility specialists most commonly treat with drugs originate in the ovaries. In my own practice, I've discovered that biopsies taken from malfunctioning ovaries frequently indicate bacterial infection. This fact alone makes me even more confident in my recommendation that antibiotic therapy should be a patient's first choice, before resorting to more toxic medications. It may turn out that this first choice is the only therapeutic choice a patient will have to make.

For some women, drug treatment may indeed prove to be the final answer to reversing an infertile situation caused by poor ovarian function, but that happy ending does not come without risks. The ovary is particularly vulnerable to bad side effects from fertility drugs, including hyperstimulation syndrome (during which the ovary may grow from the size of an almond to the size of a fist or even larger), ovarian-cyst formation, bleeding disorders, and ovarian rupture, which can lead to all sorts of pelvic disasters.

While drug-related complications rarely become this serious, they are well worth avoiding altogether, and that is why I so strongly advocate seeing what antibiotic therapy can do first. Maybe it won't go all the way to restoring fertility, at least within the desired time frame, but maybe it will help fertility drugs perform more safely and effectively. That's what happened with Sharon, who endured eight miscarriages between 1984 and 1988 before she became my patient at the age of thirty-four.

Sharon's first miscarriage ended her only spontaneous pregnancy. The remaining seven miscarriages occurred while she was undergoing different courses of drug therapy administered by other fertility specialists. The first four of these failed pregnancies were stimulated with clomiphene; the last three, with Pergonal. The therapeutic goal had always been the same: to stimulate her ovaries so they would produce eggs, nourish them to maturity, release them at the proper time, and finally, keep up a steady supply of progesterone to the uterine lining.

When I first examined Sharon, shortly after her eighth miscarriage, she was ovulating very irregularly. She was also panic-stricken at the prospect of suffering premature menopause. "I'm willing to do anything," she told me. "I'm not afraid of trying something more radical."

Ironically, I felt Sharon's situation called for something much simpler. It was obvious to me that her drug treatments and the subsequent pregnancies had steadily eroded the health of her ovaries, and I suspected a progressively worsening bacterial infection might be primarily responsible for her troubles.

Sharon and her husband both tested positive for anaerobic bacteria: three different types in her and two in her husband, with one shared anaerobe. I immediately put them on ten days of intravenous antibiotic therapy. Each received a combination clindamycin-gentamicin course: four doses of 900 milligrams of clindamycin were administered daily using an ambulatory pump system in a continuous infusion; the gentamicin level was adjusted on the basis of repeated blood sampling so the level of medication in the bloodstream remained in a therapeutic range.

As fate would have it, Sharon's therapy did not bring back normal ovulation after three months, at which time she was desperate to have a child. Despite this disappointment, I was sufficiently pleased with the improved hormonal function of her ovaries to think Pergonal could now be beneficial.

I started Sharon's treatment regimen with clomiphene given from day 2 through day 4 of her cycle. Then the Pergonal injections began—150 units daily for a five-day period. At the end of that period, sonography showed her ovaries were still not adequately stimulated, so Pergonal injections were given for an additional three days. On the thirteenth day of her cycle, a second sonogram documented three well-formed eggs, two in the right ovary and one in the left ovary. An HCG injection was administered, and the couple was instructed as to the best timing for sexual intercourse. The very first month brought about a pregnancy, and nine months later, in June of 1989, Sharon gave birth to a healthy daughter.

I sincerely believe that if we'd let nature take its course for two or three years after the antibiotic therapy, Sharon would have become pregnant spontaneously, and her pregnancy would have been a similarly fortunate one. A fertility drug, however, enabled Sharon and her husband to have their child at the time that was best for them. And antibiotic therapy, I am sure, provided much better circumstances in which that drug could do its intended job.

Men

Because the same hormones that induce egg development in a woman also induce sperm development in a man, it is not surprising that specialists use the same fertility drugs to rectify both male and female hormonal imbalances. For men, however, there is really only one reproductive problem that may respond favorably to fertility-drug treatment: a low sperm count (oligo-spermia) due to insufficient hormone production by the pituitary gland.

Other male reproductive problems that often appear together with a low sperm count are poor sperm motility (that is, the sperm do not move as swiftly or efficiently as they should) and/or poor sperm morphology (the sperm have structural irregularities that impede their ability to swim or impregnate an egg). Sometimes these two problems clear up as a side effect of increasing the sperm count. Overcoming them directly, whether or not the patient has a low sperm count as well, is best considered in the context of artificial insemination and in vitro fertilization. (See my discussion of assisted reproduction, below.)

When fertility specialists detect a low sperm count in a patient who does not have a varicocele, they can't help suspecting the pituitary gland is at fault, since the hormonal output of the pituitary gland raises the testosterone level in the testicles, which, in turn, stimulates the manufacture of sperm. Fertility drugs attempt to compensate for a presumably malfunctioning pituitary gland by working directly on the testicles to boost the testosterone level.

When the problem is mild, many doctors rely on clomiphene. Typically, a patient will be put on a three- to six-month course of 25 milligrams a day for twenty-five days per month. On occasion, clomiphene can stimulate a man's sperm production, but I don't know of a single case where administering clomiphene to a man has been solely responsible for reversing a couple's infertility.

In more serious cases (for example, when the sperm count is especially low, or when a low count is accompanied by abnormally small testicles), treatment with HCG and Pergonal is often administered. The HCG stimulates testosterone production. A patient may be given two or three injections a week for five to six months until his testosterone level is acceptable. At that time, Pergonal is usually added to the patient's regular HCG injections in order to escalate his sperm production. In general, however, there is a very low rate of response.

In my own practice, I am very reluctant to use fertility drugs to create a higher sperm count. Many of my cases have indicated that a patient's low sperm count does not necessarily or entirely result from poor pituitary performance (a condition that is difficult to prove and easy to assume); instead, a low count may be due exclusively or primarily to bacterial infection in the testes.

What I've said before bears repeating: fertility drugs are quite potent and can easily throw a reproductive system out of whack; therefore, antibiotic therapy—which is very promising and far less toxic—should take precedence.

At any rate, I could never justify artificially increasing the number of sperm a man produces without first making sure his reproductive system isn't contaminated by bacteria. Otherwise, I would only be increasing the chances for him to infect or re-infect his partner.

.... SURGERY ....

Any form of surgery on the male or female genital tract to enhance the possibility of reproduction is, to my mind, a definite second-tier strategy. No matter what good it may accomplish or how certain a therapist may be that it is the only solution, reproductive surgery is a radical and risky invasion of a highly delicate system. Before any kind of reproductive surgery is undertaken, the system must at least be free of bacterial infection. Otherwise, surgery could inadvertently cause the infection to spread, either by means of the procedure itself or by means of the structural changes it creates. Assuming the system does prove to be infected and the infection is cleared, then if it's at all possible and appropriate, surgery should be delayed until it can be determined whether the newly bacteria-free system is also a newly fertile one.

In examining drug therapies, we started with a woman's point of view. Since we've just considered low sperm count and since this problem lies behind 80 percent of the cases involving surgery on the male reproductive system, we'll begin the examination of surgical therapies from a man's point of view.

Men

Approximately 10 percent of all men and 40 percent of men who visit fertility clinics have a swollen (or varicose) vein on their left testicle. As I mentioned in Chapter 2, this kind of vein, a varicocele, can impede sperm production by raising the temperature in the testicles.

The standard treatment for varicoceles is surgery, in which the vein is cut and stitched. A less conventional but increasingly popular surgical procedure is called balloon occlusion. A silicone balloon, inserted into the vein through a catheter, is left there to block off the blood supply. Although this latter approach is quicker, easier, and less painful, it is also riskier; the balloon may loosen and float elsewhere in the body, causing serious blood clots. In either case, there's at least a 15- to 20-percent chance that a varicocele will recur.

For those who are afraid of surgical intervention, a newly invented testicular-cooling device is available. This device is best described as a pair of modified jockey shorts with a coolant circulating in the fabric that intimately surrounds the testicles. The device can lower the testicular core temperature to the desired level. Thus, if a man can accept the discomfort of wearing the device for a three-month period, he may be able to avoid surgery, except if he desires a longer-lasting correction of his infertile situation.

In my opinion, varicocele surgery is performed far too soon in many cases and far too often in general. Usually, it's the first, if not the only, course of action advised. The operation may well yield a satisfyingly fast solution for the varicocele itself, but is it the best possible way to restore the couple's fertility? In other words, is it in the best interest of the patient, his partner, and even the child they may bear?

I think not. First, the man's genital tract should be cleared of bacterial infection. This step alone may take care of the existing infertility problem, which may or may not be low sperm production. Assuming antibiotic therapy does not take care of that problem, then, and only then, would I advise surgery. Surgery before clearing up any possible infection is irresponsible for reasons I've already stated: if surgery provides a bacterially contaminated man with more and/or better-functioning sperm, then he is all the more capable of passing along his infection to his wife and, through her, to their yet-to-be-born child.

A varicocele may be the sole cause of a couple's infertility if the man has never fathered a child and if the two partners are otherwise healthy. Let's say the couple has produced a child within the past couple of years, however—a very common scenario. Faced with this history, I would not automatically assume the man's varicocele is to blame for their current infertility, and I would argue against an operation to correct it unless all other possible causes were ruled out. In my opinion, it is far more likely the couple's infertility is the result of a growing bacterial infection in the woman's reproductive tract dating from her previous pregnancy.

The varicocele condition no doubt plays a role in the scenario I've just mentioned. The elevated temperature in the scrotum increases the amount of harmful bacteria in the man's system, intensifying his contamination of his partner so much that she becomes incapable of sustaining another pregnancy. I find it extremely difficult to believe, however, that a varicocele condition by itself could have affected the quality and quantity of the man's sperm adversely enough in only two years to render conception impossible.

Accordingly, whenever I interview a patient with a varicocele condition, I always look for signs of secondary infertility in the couple's history:

• Did the woman notice any change in her period after the birth of her previous child?

- Did she experience any pain or discomfort in her genital tract or in her abdominal region in general?

- Did she develop any of the major PMS symptoms? (See Chapter 5.)

- Is the couple's child frequently sick or ill-behaved?

If I can establish a reasonable case for secondary infertility through history taking and culture studies, I put off any consideration of varicocele surgery until antibiotic therapy has been given every chance to restore the health of each partner's reproductive system.

Antibiotic therapy alone worked for Bernard and Carol. They came to me in the summer of 1989, after they had been trying unsuccessfully for several months to conceive a second child (their daughter was two years old at the time). After I reviewed the questionnaire and examined Bernard, the three of us discussed their therapeutic options. I explained that I suspected bacterial infection as the prime culprit. In addition to the presence of a varicocele on Bernard's testicle, their reproductive history included Carol's having several bouts of vaginitis shortly after giving birth.

Carol and Bernard agreed to be cultured, and I found chlamydia in both of them. They immediately consented to the six-week antibiotic regimen my laboratory recommends for a chlamydia genital-tract infection. That treatment consists of 100 milligrams of doxycycline three times daily for three weeks, followed by 333 milligrams of erythromycin four times a day for three weeks.

As soon as I was satisfied that both Carol's and Bernard's reproductive systems were uncontaminated, I advised them to try unprotected intercourse again. In two months, Carol was pregnant, and right now, that pregnancy is in its fourth, trouble-free month.

Many couples have come to me after a varicocele operation has failed to restore their fertility. In February 1986, Jeanette read about my antibiotic therapy in a popular magazine and encouraged her husband, Carl, to join her in consulting me. A year previously, another specialist attributed their primary infertility to Carl's varicocele. Carl had it surgically corrected, but they remained infertile. A second specialist advised Prednisone—a cortisone-like drug—as therapy for sperm antibodies. This tactic didn't help either.

I tested Carl and Jeanette for bacteria and found five anaerobes and chlamydia in Carl and four matching anaerobes and chlamydia in Jeanette, plus sperm antibodies. Evidently her prior therapy succeeded in suppressing her antibodies only temporarily. For the chlamydia infection, I prescribed three weeks of doxycycline followed by erythromycin; for the anaerobic bacteria, I continued the treatment with two additional weeks of Flagyl, 500 milligrams four times daily. By June 1986, Jeanette was free of bacterial infection. By October, the sperm antibodies had disappeared. Over the next two years, she had two normal pregnancies resulting in two healthy sons.

My hesitancy to advise surgery for varicoceles stems from a fundamental preference to avoid such a traumatic procedure as surgery, no matter what form it may take, unless it is absolutely necessary. This is not to say varicocele repair can't make a critical difference in a couple's ability to have a child; many times, it can. The experience of Gail and Evan, two of my current patients, offers a good illustration.

As soon as Gail and Evan were married, Gail became pregnant. Three months later, she miscarried; they remained child-less for the next five years. I diagnosed Gail as having luteal-phase defect associated with endometriosis. Evan had a varicocele and a very low sperm count. In this case, I suspected both partners were suffering from bacterial infection but that Evan's varicocele was, by now, directly responsible for his low sperm count. First, I tested them for bacteria and found myco-plasma and three anaerobes in each culture. Next, I placed them on a three-week doxycycline course (100 milligrams three times daily) followed by a two-week Flagyl course (500 milli-grams four times daily). When I was finally convinced both partners were free of bacteria and that Gail's reproductive sys-tem was fully restored to health, I recommended surgery for Evan's varicocele. One year after the surgery, Gail delivered a seven-pound boy.

Women

For women, recent advances in surgical procedures to cor-rect genital-tract problems have achieved miracles. In the late 1960s, the advent of microsurgery—operations featuring mi-croscopes and microscopic knives, forceps, needles, and threads—enabled specially trained surgeons to perform all sorts of delicate repairs they couldn't do, or couldn't do nearly as well, before, including excising small adhesions and reshaping intricate malformations in the uterus, the fallopian tubes, and the ovaries. Beginning in 1979, their work was made even more effective by the introduction of microsurgery via laparoscopy, in which surgical intruments or even laser beams are passed through thin operating tubes under laparoscopic visualization.

But while reproductive surgery has become vastly more far-reaching and sophisticated, it still remains invasive and potentially dangerous. And while, in some cases, it can make the difference between being fertile and being infertile, it is among the last steps to be considered, not the first.

Too often, the reverse happens. Aside from the small number of unscrupulous doctors who steer their patients toward surgery for the money it will bring, there are many doctors who are so fascinated with the new technological advances that they advise immediate surgery for every applicable situation, knowing it will "do the trick" quickly and impressively. Many patients, all too eager to believe that their uncooperative bodies, like broken-down machines, can be fixed with tools, accept this advice without question.

Given the inherent danger and expense of surgery, not to mention its capacity to spread infection, I recommend opting for a medical approach whenever possible. My feeling in this matter is especially strong if the reproductive problem seems to be attributable to adhesions in the peritoneal cavity or around the fallopian tubes—the situations for which surgery is most commonly prescribed. Most adhesions of this type are caused by bacterial infection ascending from the vagina.

Since most patients diagnosed as having pelvic adhesions can't recall an episode that could be considered the beginning of the process, it is logical to assume their adhesions developed as the result of bacterial irritation over an extended period of time. It is also logical to assume the same bacterial irritation is still actively working against the local tissue. Therefore, I believe such cases require broad-spectrum antiobiotic therapy directed primarily against anaerobic bacteria.

In October of 1987, Joy decided the time was right to conceive a child with her present husband, Ralph. Having had genital-tract problems during a previous marriage, she wanted to be sure everything was OK before she and Ralph stopped using condoms, so she went to a fertility specialist in Boston, where they'd just moved. She told the specialist that she had had an induced abortion in 1983. In the months that followed, she had experienced progressively worse pains in the abdomen, which had been attributed at the time to PID and had been treated with oral drugs.

After listening to Joy's history, the Boston specialist performed a laparoscopy and discovered a group of fairly large adhesions behind the uterus and a few fine adhesions around the right fallopian tube and ovary. He proceeded to burn away the adhesions with laser surgery. Since no pregnancy occurred afterward, however, a friend convinced her to see me for a second opinion; and so, in January 1988, she made the trip to my Manhattan laboratory.

When Joy told me her complete reproductive history, I theorized her first husband had been the source of a bacterial infection that had spread through her genital tract during her pregnancy and had caused the PID she had experienced after that pregnancy was aborted. Fortunately, she was able to provide me with a videotape of the laparoscopy that her Boston specialist had performed. When I saw the adhesions, my theory turned into a tentative conclusion. I believed a bacterial infection had created those adhesions and, since no broad-spectrum antibiotic was given following surgery, that the harmful bacteria were still present in her reproductive system.

Joy's culture did, in fact, reveal two anaerobes. Ralph's culture revealed none. I advised Joy to undergo ten days of intravenous clindamycin and gentamicin medication (administered by pump so she could go about her normal daily routines). When the ten days were over, I performed a "second look" laparoscopy. Comparing her present condition with the condition I had seen previously on the videotape, I realized that the pelvic damage she had sustained from her infection was beyond repair. At this point, both her fallopian tubes were badly involved in a complicated web of adhesions, and when we attempted to peruse the tubes with a marker dye, the delicate fingers at the ends of the tubes were so swollen they refused to pass the dye.

I concluded that the surgery performed by Joy's previous specialist had only accelerated her infection. Now, the best recommendation I could make for Joy was to pursue in vitro fertilization. On her second attempt, she became pregnant, and today, she and Ralph are the proud parents of twin girls.

Not all adhesions in a woman's reproductive system are caused by bacterial infection. Some are the result of advanced endometriosis; others may be scars from previous pelvic surgery (like an appendectomy or an operation on the bowels). While these latter types account for a very small percentage of adhesions, surgery is advisable if such adhesions do seem to be responsible for a couple's infertility. Before surgery, however, the patient should be checked for bacterial infection, and any existing infection needs to be eradicated. If this isn't done, when the adhesions are surgically severed or burned, blood oozing from the adhesions will provide a fertile milieu for spreading bacteria, and new, bacteria-caused adhesions may form as soon as a week or two later. The problem is much worse, of course, if the original adhesions were full of bacteria in the first place.

Today, many specialists prescribe ten days of doxycycline treatment after reproductive surgery. From the standpoint of proper antibiotic therapy in such a situation, this treatment is woefully inadequate. The only safe, healthy, and reliable approach to a bacterial infection of any kind anywhere in the female or the male genital tract is to get rid of the infection first; then, move on to whatever other measures need to be taken to facilitate a pregnancy.

.... ASSISTED REPRODUCTION ....

So far, we've examined treatments for restoring the reproductive health of both the male and the female partner so they can go about having a baby in a natural way. Occasionally, however, an infertility problem can't be solved. When couples face this dilemma, they may need outside help in getting a pregnancy started.

There are two major categories of assisted reproduction: artificial insemination and in vitro fertilization. I'll address each one separately in the light of what antibiotic therapy can do.

Artificial Insemination

Although artificial insemination is commonly thought to be a twentieth-century, ultrascientific approach to overcoming infertility, it's actually one of the oldest recorded techniques in history. Egyptian papyruses mention it. So does the Talmud. But for millennia (as far as we know), it took only one form: the transfer of freshly released sperm into the vagina.

Historical evidence also suggests artificial insemination was used in only two situations. Sometimes, the would-be father was too inhibited to ejaculate inside or in sight of the would-be mother. More often, the woman was unable to conceive by the man in the normal manner and was forbidden or unwilling to have intercourse with anyone else, which necessitated a nonintimate arrangement with another male. In either case, semen was collected outside her body and quickly injected into her—by reed, tube, or plunger.

These reasons for artificial insemination continue to exist; but modern breakthroughs in identifying the causes of infertility, in collecting and storing sperm, and in administering sperm into a woman's reproductive system have greatly increased the range of potential applications for artificial insemination. Still, as always, the most commonly prescribed treatment for dealing with male-factor infertility problems, artificial insemination today is also helpful in working around certain female-factor infertility problems and in making it possible for a couple to conceive a child at a time of their choosing, regardless of whether the father is present or capable at that particular time.

First, let's look at male-related issues. Aside from impotence or a performance problem, the main reasons a man may have difficulty impregnating his partner—according to most doctors—are a low sperm count, poor sperm motility, and/or poor sperm morphology. Given these conditions, the man's sperm can be specially processed and artificially inseminated so their chances of fertilizing an egg are greatly enhanced.

The principal form of sperm processing to compensate for a low sperm count is called sperm washing. The ejaculate, suspended in a culture medium, is spun in a centrifuge, which separates the sperm itself from the seminal fluid. The concentrated sperm are then injected into the woman's genital tract.

In cases of poor sperm motility or morphology, a swim-up process is used, whereby sperm (unwashed or washed) literally swim up a tube of culture medium. The best swimmers—the ones that reach the top of the tube first—are captured and inseminated.

For women, the major infertility problem currently overcome by artificial insemination is the presence of hostile cervical mucus. In this situation, the sperm is injected directly into the uterus (a process known as intrauterine insemination, or IUI), thus bypassing the cervix altogether. If the uterine milieu is also hostile to sperm, then sperm can be injected directly into the fallopian tubes (a process known as intratubal insemination, or ITI). These different placement options are also serviceable in cases of a woman's partner having a low sperm count, poor sperm motility, or poor sperm morphology. Sperm that are injected directly into the uterus or the fallopian tubes have a far shorter distance to swim to the eggs.

Perhaps the most beneficial modern-day advance in artificial insemination has been the ability to freeze sperm so they can be used at a later date. Some couples choose to freeze a sample of the male partner's sperm so the female partner has the opportunity to conceive his child no matter what happens—an extended separation, an event that might render the male physically incapable of fathering a child (such as a severe groin injury or the effects of chemotherapy), or even his death. Other couples, who can't conceive because of problems with the male partner's sperm or who don't want to risk reproducing some genetic defect in the male partner's line, choose among frozen and "typed" sperm specimens donated to a sperm bank by other men.

I am entirely sympathetic to the use of artificial insemination in these latter situations involving insurmountable barriers in time and circumstance. I also feel it is a justified treatment whenever a man has an intransigent performance problem but can still masturbate to a climax or whenever the volume of semen is so small it gets completely lost in the walls of the vagina. Otherwise, I think fertility specialists misunderstand and abuse artificial insemination more than any other single therapy.

As I've already discussed in this chapter, antibiotic therapy alone may reverse an infertile situation that is apparently caused by a low sperm count, poor sperm motility, or poor sperm morphology. If, in fact, testicular infection is playing havoc with sperm production, the right combination of antibiotics will knock the infection out. In any event, antibiotic therapy will strip the sperm of any harmful bacteria they may be carrying into the woman's genital tract, and such an infection in itself may well be the real cause of the couple's infertility. Hostile cervical mucus can also be successfully treated with antibiotic therapy, and it should be treated instead of merely avoided.

Unfortunately, the process of washing sperm does not remove any harmful bacteria that may be adhering to them. Artificially inseminating a woman with washed sperm that have not been tested for bacteria—and treated if necessary—is, in my opinion, courting disaster. Using IUI or ITI to bypass hostile cervical mucus without first making every attempt, beginning with antibiotic therapy, to render that mucus hospitable, is, I believe, similarly dangerous.

At best, with no other problems to be managed besides insufficient or poorly performing sperm, artificial insemination has about a 20-percent chance of causing a pregnancy. This is not a high enough success rate to warrant the current emphasis on artificial insemination within the profession. At worst, it can wind up giving the recipient a bacterial infection that endangers her health, any subsequent pregnancy, and the well-being of any child or children that she brings into the world. In aiming for the best, a fertility program involving artificial insemination must first involve testing and, if appropriate, therapy to make sure there are no harmful bacteria attached to the sperm or preexisting in the woman's reproductive system.

In Vitro Fertilization

Simply speaking, in vitro (Latin for "in a glass") fertilization is a three-step process:

1. Eggs are surgically removed from the ovary.

2. Eggs are fertilized with sperm in a special culture dish.

3. Fertilized eggs are surgically placed in the uterus, where it is hoped they will implant so a normal pregnancy can begin.

As practiced, however, in vitro fertilization is anything but simple. It's a very complicated, uncertain, and expensive process, and the specific form it takes can vary considerably from case to case.

A woman who is unable to produce healthy eggs may require heavy doses of fertility drugs ahead of time. If the man's sperm are poor performers, the woman's eggs may need to be drilled (a recently developed form of microsurgery known as partial

101

zona dissection) to make sperm penetration easier in the culture dish. For couples who, apparently, have no one serious reproductive problem but still can't conceive, gamete intrafallopian transfer (or GIFT) may be advised. This is an extremely sophisticated microsurgical procedure in which the eggs and the sperm are mixed together inside the fallopian tube so fertilization has a better chance of occurring "naturally."

In vitro fertilization can definitely be a godsend for women whose fallopian tubes are completely dysfunctional or missing (although a tube compromised by bacterial infection can often regenerate within six to ten months after antibiotic therapy). Generally, however, in vitro fertilization is prescribed far more frequently than it should be. Many conditions that prompt specialists to recommend it, such as sperm-antibody problems, endometriosis, or a dry cervical milieu, can be corrected fairly easily with other, less costly and less time-consuming therapies. And the success rate for in vitro fertilization is discouragingly low. On a national average, 85 percent of in vitro patients fail to get pregnant; a mere 7 percent end up giving birth to a live baby.

Why, then, is in vitro fertilization such a popular therapy? The most plausible reason is that in vitro fertilization enables both patients and their doctors to bypass months and maybe even years of experimentation with other therapies. The body is causing complications? Let's try something else altogether! The "bad" reason is that in vitro fertilization involves a great deal of money. Many patients truly believe that the more money they spend on their infertility problem, the greater the chance they have of solving it. Some doctors are all too willing to encourage this belief for their personal benefit or for the benefit of their clinic.

Assuming in vitro fertilization is essential for a couple to have a child, prior antibiotic therapy can raise the odds that it will be successful. Failed attempts at in vitro fertilization can often be attributed to bacterially infected eggs or to a bacterially infected uterine lining, which proves incapable of holding onto the fertilized egg after it is surgically inserted. Antibiotic therapy can eliminate these problems, plus it can help the entire reproductive system to function more efficiently throughout the pregnancy. In my own practice, antibiotic therapy always precedes in vitro fertilization, and I am extremely proud to say that my antibiotic-treated patients' success rate for in-vitro-related pregnancy and live birth is slightly more than twice the norm.

For Ronnie, in vitro fertilization was, quite appropriately, the last-resort strategy in a long, complex, and exhausting case. Ronnie was a DES baby, and I suspect her genital-tract contamination came from her mother. After Ronnie married Ted in 1979, she relied on the Dalkon shield IUD for birth control and began suffering pelvic pains within the very first month of use.

Looking back, I believe these pains signaled the onset of a serious bacterial infection. I can't be certain whether this infection came from bacteria in Ted's seminal fluid—bacteria that used the IUD as an opportunistic device to "wick" farther into Ronnie's system—or whether it came from her own vertically transmitted bacteria, which were pushed into her upper reproductive system when the IUD was inserted. Whichever way the infection developed, Ronnie didn't have any idea what was happening. At the end of her first year of marriage, she went off birth control to have a baby, and the result was an ectopic pregnancy.

Ronnie and Ted sought my help five childless years later, and

103

I reconstructed much of the history I have just recited from the information they gave me during our first conference. Certain that an infected fallopian tube (due to PID) was the direct cause of her ectopic pregnancy, I evaluated Ted and Ronnie for bacterial contamination and found three shared anaerobes in their cultures.

If a woman has had one ectopic pregnancy, she faces a five to eight times greater likelihood of having another ectopic pregnancy in the remaining tube because it, too, is apt to be infected. To reduce this risk for Ronnie and Ted, I put both of them on a two-week course of intravenous clindamycin and gentamicin. Afterward, I performed a hysterosalpingogram to help determine the health of Ronnie's remaining tube. According to the evidence, the tube still had a chance of functioning properly. Therefore, I advised Ronnie and Ted to resume their attempt to achieve a pregnancy, but I also recommended we follow Ronnie's progress closely if and when a pregnancy began.

Two months later, Ronnie reported to my laboratory five days after she missed her period. I decided to perform a beta subunit (BSU) pregnancy test. The beta subunit is part of a pregnancy hormone produced by the placenta, the concentration of which doubles every two or three days during pregnancy. Pregnancies conceived in a fallopian tube do not initially thrive as well as normal pregnancies, and thus a delay in BSU production is the most sensitive indicator of a misplaced pregnancy. Two tests of Ronnie's blood conducted one week apart revealed an unusually low rise in the level of BSU, and so I advised a sonogram to see where the fetus was positioned.

Sadly, this pregnancy, too, was ectopic, despite the fact that we'd considerably reduced the risk. A laparotomy (a surgical operation through the abdomen) was unable to save Ronnie's remaining tube, but it did reveal the full extent of the damage caused by her pelvic infection. It was now apparent both tubes had been rendered irreversibly incapable of delivering a fertilized egg to the uterus.

I advised another set of culture studies for Ronnie and Ted, and when one anaerobe reappeared in both samples, I put them on a second, two-week course of intravenous therapy. Then they entered an in vitro fertilization program. They conceived in their first trial, and subsequently Ronnie delivered healthy twins.

Many patients seek my help when in vitro fertilization has failed to work for them. Beverly and Philip consulted me after two unsuccessful in vitro trials. Both of Beverly's tubes were irreparably blocked, so this last-tier, last-block therapy was their only hope. Beverly got right to the point in our first interview: "We're counting on you to make in vitro work."

After hearing Beverly and Philip's history, I could deduce that bacteria attached to Philip's sperm (which were still "good performers") had infected Beverly and that the infection had developed into PID. This disease had not only ruined her tubes, but it was also preventing her from sustaining a pregnancy begun by in vitro fertilization. When I tested them and found two anaerobes and chlamydia in each culture, I prescribed ten days of intravenous antibiotic therapy.

Normally, I would counsel couples in such a situation to let six months pass after bacteria have been cleared from their systems before trying in vitro fertilization again. But because Beverly was already forty-two years old, I suggested only a three-month wait. The first trial worked, and nine months later, I delivered a healthy boy.

Later, Beverly wrote me a note saying, "My husband and I

especially appreciated the fact that you listened carefully to us and took a more thorough history than we had encountered elsewhere. You really gave thought to what we were telling you, and had a positive, activist, scientific approach that worked for us." I quote her letter because it draws attention to the most important aspect of any infertility therapy—particularly one that involves such a complicated process as in vitro fertilization: namely, the need to enlist a couple's cooperation in examining their past and present reproductive experiences closely and critically so the best possible therapeutic program can be devised to meet their particular situation.

The final case I'd like to share in this chapter illustrates a fairly frequent and always happy occurrence in my practice: the discovery that in vitro fertilization, previously claimed to be the one and only potential solution to a couple's infertility problem, is, instead, not necessary at all. Germaine and Stan tried for three years to have a child without ever conceiving. None of the fertility specialists they consulted could find anything wrong with them. Each specialist eventually gave up testing and suggested in vitro fertilization, which, unfortunately, is a common prescription when the cause of a couple's infertility can't be identified.

By the time friends referred Stan and Germaine to me, they had been through three unsuccessful attempts at in vitro fertilization. At this point, they were understandably pessimistic about their chances of success a fourth time around. Germaine confessed to me, "We hadn't planned on re-applying for in vitro, but then we heard about your therapy. We decided it was worth seeing if it would make a difference."

I tested both of them and found the same three anaerobes in Germaine's cervical culture and Stan's semen. After ten days of intravenous antibiotic treatment, I tested them again, and the anaerobes were gone. At thirty-four, Germaine was still relatively young. I advised them to put off the next in vitro trial at least six months so her reproductive system would have plenty of time to recover from any damage the infection may have caused. Because they wanted to take advantage of a sudden vacation opportunity, they wound up postponing that next trial two additional months. While they were on vacation, they achieved pregnancy spontaneously. That was two years ago. Today, they have two children: a fifteen-month-old daughter and a six-week-old son.

I can't prove beyond any shadow of a doubt that antibiotic treatment made it possible for Germaine and Stan to have a baby. At the moment, given all the uncertainties that surround the why's and wherefore's of pregnancy in general, let alone the specific mysteries of cases like the one I just described, medical science doesn't offer any means for establishing such proof. What I can say with complete conviction, however, is that antibiotic treatment is the only fertility therapy that works to restore the natural health of male and female genital tracts, and if the reproductive systems of both would-be parents are free of bacterial infection, each is much better equipped to function as it was designed to function.

Chapter 5

....

Beyond Conception:
Other Effective Applications of Antibiotic Therapy

For most people, the pelvic area is a dark, mysterious netherworld. Messy, awkward, and troublesome processes take place there that upset our equilibrium and that our upbringing trains us to ignore. The nervous system may register all sorts of ambiguous sensations from the pelvic area—queasiness, strain, pressure, itchiness, soreness, burning, or cramping—but the brain usually shuns thinking about them.

Often, however, a signal from the pelvic area becomes so strong it's incapacitating. In a man's case, the most common symptom of this type is an excruciating pain whenever he urinates, possibly accompanied by a strange discharge from the penis. In a woman's case, a variety of intense symptoms are possible, befitting the greater extent and complexity of her genital tract. A chronic irritation in her vagina may make it impossible for her to enjoy sexual intercourse. A swollen and tender abdomen may destroy her ability to concentrate on her work.

By the time a pelvic signal is this pronounced, the problem behind the signal may be far advanced. In addition to jeopardizing the victim's ability to parent a child, it may even threaten his or her life. Tragically, many equally critical problems never do announce themselves. Instead, they continue to worsen, not only from their lack of detection but also from our partly unintentional, partly willful ignorance and neglect of what can happen "down there."

111

In my practice, I use antibiotic therapy to treat many bacteria-related reproductive health problems besides infertility, from relatively simple ones like vaginitis and prostatitis to complex ones like PMS and PID. Although each of these conditions can be a precursor to full-blown infertility, they are all illnesses in their own right. Many of the people who come to my laboratory to be treated for these illnesses—or to be treated so that these illnesses won't develop—are not interested in having children, at least not right away. Instead, they're concerned about their own well-being. In this chapter, I'll discuss the major reproductive problems short of infertility and how my therapy works to restore health.

CHLAMYDIA: FIGHTING THE .... PHANTOM ....

Today, the fastest-growing and most prevalent sexually transmitted disease (STD) is chlamydia infection. In the United States alone, there are over 4.5 million newly reported cases of chlamydia infection each year, compared to one million cases of gonorrhea (the second highest STD). Among the population at large, one out of every ten people is suspected of harboring this troublesome bacterium in his or her genital tract.

Perhaps chlamydia infection has always been the most prevalent STD. If so, the chlamydia bacterium has certainly done its damage in the dark. Prior to the late 1970s, it was familiar to medical science only as the cause of conjunctivitis (or eye inflammation). Doctors were aware that a newborn could develop conjunctivitis after having been exposed to chlamydia in the mother's genital tract, but they did not associate it with infection of the genital tract itself, nor did they consider that it might be transmitted sexually.

Now, thanks to the invention of more sensitive testing procedures, we know chlamydia is the reigning monarch among STDs. I also believe, as I stated in Chapter 3, that chlamydia infections in the genital tract can result from vertical transmission.

Whichever way the chlamydia is transmitted to its victim, the results can be disastrous. Not only is its potential for devastation so vast, but it also operates so insidiously. Gonorrheal and syphilitic infections produce gross symptoms fairly quickly; only about 10 percent of the time are these infections asymptomatic for long periods of time. Chlamydia infections, by contrast, are asymptomatic throughout in an estimated 65 percent of all cases.

In men, chlamydia can move through the genital tract like a stealth bomber, progressively causing irritation and swelling of the urethra (urethritis), the prostate (prostatitis), the epididymis (epididymitis), and finally, the testes (orchitis). When symptoms do appear, they include "burning" during urination, itching, watery discharge, and more rarely, a scrotum that is visibly (if not painfully) swollen. A case of chlamydia infection so far advanced that it affects the immune system in general may produce secondary symptoms, such as joint pain (arthritis) and painful swelling of the eye (conjunctivitis).

The appropriate treatment for a chlamydia infection is a comprehensive, high-dosage antibiotic program as soon as possible. If the infection isn't wiped out early in its history, it's very difficult later to get rid of it entirely. Consider the case of Derek, who sought my advice in 1988 for an infection that had been plaguing him since 1985.

Derek owns an international company and frequently spends long periods of time abroad on business. He told me he first noticed a transparent, slightly viscous discharge from his urethra shortly after a visit to one of Bangkok's infamous massage parlors. A urologist in Thailand diagnosed the problem as a chlamydia infection. Whether or not Derek picked up that infection during his massage is a moot point. He was lucky to have a symptomatic alert and a rationale for seeking help. He was unlucky, however, in his initial therapy. After the recommended course of treatment, he was fine for a few days, but as soon as he returned to the United States, the symptoms flared up again.

Derek went to a new urologist, who, like his Thai counterpart, told him he had a chlamydia infection and prescribed the "standard" ten-day course of oral tetracycline. When that didn't work, the very same program was stubbornly repeated. Again, his symptoms returned within a few days, even more virulent than they had been before. By now, urinating was always acutely painful for Derek, and the discharge was about twice as copious. "I was so frustrated," he admitted, "that I was sure that the problem was something else, something more serious than what the two doctors had told me."

Determined as he was, Derek went to a third urologist and demanded that he do everything possible to get to the bottom of his problem. The urologist advised a cystoscopy. Hearing this from Derek, I was quite bothered. Whatever pressure Derek may have been exerting as a patient, the urologist had extremely little justification for suggesting this relatively invasive procedure. A cystoscopy is a surgically facilitated explora-

tion of the genital tract designed to establish the possible presence of cancer or a polyp. In a young man (Derek was then
twenty-five years old), the symptoms he presented almost always point to bacterial infection, and every possible means of
investigating such an infection should have been tried first.

Understandably, the cystoscopy did not reveal anything suspicious. The urologist stopped there—once more, failing to
pursue other, more appropriate forms of testing. He put Derek
on four months of sulfa drugs, a somewhat blind approach to
Derek's problem, and the two of them hoped for the best. They
hoped in vain. Derek's symptoms came and went from month
to month. On the average, nothing changed.

Finally, Derek's girlfriend brought him to me. A meticu-
lously thorough analysis of his semen showed the chlamydia
was still present, aided and abetted by two anaerobes. This time
around, I prescribed intravenous antibiotic treatment, involving a high dosage of doxycycline. Within two weeks, he was no
longer experiencing painful urination or watery discharge. He
has remained asymptomatic ever since. More important, his
cultures show he has also stayed bacteria-free.

The prostate is a notoriously stubborn organ in the male
genital area. Due to its complex anatomical structure and relatively compromised blood flow, bacteria harbored within its
intricate globules are not easy to reach with medication. Therefore, an infection with chlamydia and/or a number of other
bacteria can be very difficult to eradicate. Chronic prostatitis
and, later on, chronic enlargement of the prostate, will lead to
urinary-flow obstruction, which necessitates a prostatectomy
(surgical removal of the prostate gland), either through the
urethra or through the abdomen. Like Derek, many of my male
patients who go through the intravenous antibiotic regimen are

not worried about infertility. Instead, they are troubled by an ever-recurring prostate inflammation that blocks urination or renders it extremely painful.

In women, chlamydia can be responsible for similarly intractable infections. Moving up through the genital tract, it can cause irritation and swelling of the vagina (vaginitis), the cervix (cervicitis), the uterine lining (endometritis), the fallopian tubes (salpingitis), and the ovary (oophoritis).

As for symptoms of chlamydia infection, they're even scarcer among women than they are among men. Over 70 percent of female victims are asymptomatic. When symptoms do appear, they are usually very subtle and easily dismissed—ranging from an itching or burning sensation in the vagina to dull aches or "tender feelings" anywhere in the pelvic area. Nevertheless, these symptoms can be persistently discomforting, and in extreme cases, they can even be debilitating.

Physical pains and problems (including infertility) are not the only possible consequences of long-term chlamydia infection in the female genital tract. Such an infection can also play havoc with a woman's emotional and psychological health, particularly in the context of her sexual relationships. The story of one of my recent patients, Michelle, offers an instructive example.

Michelle developed an unusually troublesome case of vaginitis over the first few months of her marriage to Victor. By the fifth month, they were compelled to discontinue sexual intercourse. She was desperate enough—and wealthy enough—to consult seven gynecological specialists over the next three years. None of them was able to provide lasting relief.

Meanwhile, she and Victor were constantly teetering on the verge of divorce. They went through three rounds of marriage counseling during this time. Her continual lament was "I never had problems before I slept with him." His perpetual response was "I don't have anything wrong; she needs help, not me."

When I first met Michelle, she frankly admitted she was an "emotional wreck," fearful of intimacy with her husband and, as she put it, "slightly paranoid about therapists." By this time, Victor had finally agreed to cooperate in any testing and treatment program that showed promise. Fortunately, he was impressed with what I told him about the possible benefits of antibiotic therapy.

After reviewing their separate and combined histories, I was inclined to agree that Victor was the unwitting originator of Michelle's infection. Years before their marriage, he contracted gonorrhea. He discovered it right away, and it was quickly eradicated with penicillin—a commonplace scenario. Regrettably, the penicillin had no effect on the chlamydia bacterium that was also in his reproductive system.

For some time after an individual undergoes one kind of genital-tract infection, he or she is much less resistant to other kinds of infection. And that's what happened to Victor. Inside his genital tract, gonorrhea paved the way for a rapid spread of chlamydia, which, in addition to working on its own, is a highly opportunistic organism. He never felt the effects himself. Against the odds, his wife did.

It took two courses of antibiotic treatment administered by my laboratory before Victor and Michelle could reestablish a regular pattern of sexual intercourse. Even then, Michelle's "burning" symptom didn't abate until Victor began consistently using a condom.

Summarizing this case, I must conclude the following: although the antibiotic therapy wiped out the chlamydia infection entirely, it did not get rid of all irritating agents in Victor's seminal fluid. I must also conclude that one factor strongly mitigating against a complete cure was the tremendous psychological damage Michelle endured during her four-year battle with this notoriously insidious bacteria.

It's easy to cast Victor as a villain in the situation I've just recounted, but in handling case after case where a man has unknowingly contaminated his partner, I've learned to my sorrow that Victor's behavior—counterproductive as it may be—is normal. Anyone may experience difficulty admitting he or she is a "silent" carrier of disease. Faced with taking the blame for another person's pain, most people instinctively react with disbelief, defensiveness, and denial. To make matters worse, there's the widespread lack of knowledge about genital-tract function, dysfunction, and therapy that I mentioned at the beginning of this chapter. More than any other factor, this ignorance serves to perpetuate negative attitudes about sexually related issues and, therefore, negative reproductive health situations.

To underscore these points, let me describe the history of another bacterially infected woman, Pat, whose sensitive and intelligent partner, Gary, the apparent source of contamination, turned out to be maddeningly uncooperative. In this case, the harmful organism in Pat's genital tract was not chlamydia but an anaerobe. The presenting symptom, however, was the same: a burning itch signaling vaginitis. And what happened to Pat, medically and personally, could have happened no matter what specific bacterium was involved.

Trouble started for Pat and Gary four years before they came to me, during their sophomore year in college. Prior to the onset of their sexual relationship, both had been virgins. Pat first experienced vaginal irritation within their first month of inti-macy. Five months later, her vaginitis was so far advanced that she and Gary had to discontinue having intercourse.

Gary was compassionate but, naturally, frustrated. His atti-tude worsened when a specialist told Pat, "You're allergic to your boyfriend"—a rather crude diagnosis! The specialist gave her antihistamines, but her vaginitis continued without relief. Next, the same specialist prescribed steroids to suppress her immune system so that it wouldn't generate such painful symp-toms. This therapy also failed to work.

Gary's patience and faith were steadily eroding, and he was less and less afraid of expressing his negative feelings about the "sexual problem" he and Pat were experiencing and about therapists in general. Pat, on the other hand, felt obligated to suppress her fear and guilt and to persevere as optimistically as possible in her search for a cure.

Pat's next specialist performed a colposcopy (an examination of the vagina and cervix under a low-power microscope) and saw what he described as "mild inflammation." He attributed it to a virus and sent a biopsy to four other experts for their opinion. Two of them said her trouble probably was due to a viral infection; two of them said it probably wasn't. The upshot was that Pat visited yet another specialist. This one prescribed a high dosage of Prednisone, which caused her to develop a mild psychosis.

I was Pat's fourth specialist. Gary came to my laboratory with Pat in the spirit of a vigilant skeptic rather than an open-minded collaborator (he had recently become a medical stu-dent, which only made matters worse). By now, they had been together four years. Because they swore they had been faithful to each other all that time, I conjectured that either Pat or Gary (or both) had been infected by vertically transmitted bacteria. When Gary heard that he might be at fault and, regardless, that he, too, would have to be treated, he exploded. "That's totally asinine!" he said, venting years of anger. "I can't be infected—I don't have a single, solitary symptom!"

Reluctantly, I agreed to treat Pat alone, trusting their guarantee that she and Gary would avoid unprotected intercourse. Large quantities of a suspicious anaerobe showed up in her culture, so I put her on two weeks of intravenous clindamycin and gentamicin. Her symptoms disappeared for almost three weeks but then gradually reasserted themselves.

Gary, a self-proclaimed authority on medical matters, insisted that the early success of the antibiotic therapy had been due to a placebo effect—Pat had been so primed psychologically to feel better that she actually did, for a while. It wasn't my place to tell Gary he was wrong or to suggest his misguided concern might be making Pat's life all the more difficult. Accordingly, with great forbearance, I explained to him that Pat's infection had been so severe that her recovery was no doubt assuming a sinusoidal curve. In lay language, she would suffer gradually diminishing waves of recurring symptoms. Each bout with the "burning itch," I predicted, would be a little later and a little less intense until the condition ceased entirely.

All three of us followed the next twelve months very closely. Pat's first two bouts of vaginitis were slightly over three weeks apart. The next two bouts were a full three months apart. Her last bout came six months later. Simultaneously, Pat and Gary mellowed—as individuals and as a couple. Midway through the post-therapy year, they married, and at the end of it, Gary came to my laboratory and said, "You know what? I believe you! I'm here for testing and for the therapy, if I need it."

Gary did need antibiotic therapy, and I prescribed the same therapy for him I'd given Pat. I also advised them to continue using a condom during sexual intercourse. No course of treatment for bacterial contamination is 100-percent certain, and with an infection as disruptive as Pat's had been, I didn't feel they should take any chances.

PREMENSTRUAL
.... SYNDROME ....

Unfortunately, Gary's reluctance to admit he was part of Pat's problem typifies the ambivalent response of far too many men to their female partners' reproductive difficulties—indeed, to female sexuality in general. In no other context is this more apparent than in the tendency among men to dismiss PMS as a valid physical complaint. That the controversy around PMS continues to rage also exemplifies our culture's willful blindness toward all genital-tract problems. The name itself is a model of vagueness and evasion, and the symptoms—a complex of physical, emotional, and behavioral disorders beginning in the second part of the menstrual cycle and ending soon after menstruation—are often not taken seriously. Thus, PMS is a stand-up comic's delight, immediately provoking nervous laughter as performers conjure up demeaning images of deranged harpies or self-destructive hypochondriacs.

In fact, the problems characterizing most cases of PMS are fairly mundane in themselves. They include any combination of the following maladies: breast tenderness, increased appetite, craving for food (especially food with high carbohydrate levels), abdominal bloating, fatigue, headaches, emotional instability, loss of interest in sex, depression, anxiety, restlessness, irritability, hostility, or aggression. And for all the mystery associated with PMS (part of which is certainly due to centuries of inattention), the problems it can bring are very real and very widespread in the population. Experts estimate 90 percent of women experience one or more symptoms of PMS during their reproductive years. Within this group, 30 percent endure chronic, life-disrupting symptoms, and 5 percent are seriously incapacitated on a regular basis.

Aside from making the sufferer herself uncomfortable, PMS can wreak havoc on everyone around her. The adverse behavior it generates can disrupt family life, strain friendships, and sour working relationships. Under extreme conditions, it can even lead to such tragedies as divorce, child abuse, and violent assault.

To date, the precise causes of PMS have not been conclusively proved, and so there is no definitive cure. My own professional experience, however, leads me to believe that a high percentage of PMS cases are either directly caused or aggravated by a bacterial infection in the reproductive tract— most likely an endometrial or ovarian infection.

As often happens to clinical doctors, I deduced a possible cause after stumbling upon an evident cure. Many female infertility patients whom I had treated with broad-spectrum antibiotics confessed without prompting that their PMS symptoms thereafter were significantly and permanently alleviated. I inferred from their testimony that their PMS, along with their infertility, had been reversed through exposure to the antibiotics.

Several colleagues shared my hypothesis. Together, we designed and conducted an experiment in 1986 to test whether antibiotic therapy could offer measurable and lasting relief to PMS sufferers.

Our first challenge was to locate subjects whose PMS might be linked to bacterial infection. A newspaper advertisement was used to recruit a random cross section of candidates. From these respondents, we selected only those who were otherwise healthy and who had not taken antibiotics or any other strong medication during the previous year. Next, we disqualified any candidate who could not trace the onset of her PMS symptoms (as listed above) to a particular sexual encounter, a pregnancy-related D and C, a miscarriage, an ectopic pregnancy, or childbirth—events during which bacteria would have had a chance to invade the genital tract.

Those candidates who remained were asked to evaluate their particular symptoms daily for one complete menstrual cycle, rating each symptom on a scale of zero to ten (ten being the most highly symptomatic). If the daily average sum of a candidate's symptoms during the last six days of her cycle exceeded at least twice the daily average sum of her symptoms from days 6 through 10 of her cycle, then she would be eligible for the study. This basic test, incidentally, is a good way for women in general to begin determining whether or not they may be suffering from PMS.

Ultimately, we found thirty ideal subjects, all of whom claimed that their PMS symptoms noticeably interfered with their daily social and professional activities. For the duration of the study, they agreed to avoid any other medications stronger than aspirin or acetaminophen and to maintain phone contact with us—a means of ensuring their compliance with the experimental protocol. If a subject was sexually active, her partner had to agree either to use condoms or join in the treatment regimen.

The first month of the experiment consisted of drug-free self-evaluation. Each woman kept a daily record of her symptoms, similar to the record she had kept immediately prior to the experiment, plus she filled out a detailed questionnaire regarding her menstruation: the number of days, the consistency of the flow (spotty, light, medium, heavy), the color of the flow (brown, light red, dark red) and the overall severity of pain each day of the menses (on a scale of zero to ten, with ten the most painful).

At the start of the second month, the thirty subjects, continuing to monitor their symptoms day by day, were randomly divided into two treatment groups. Each subject received a supply of 100-milligram capsules to be taken orally twice a day, but the capsules for one group contained a placebo (a neutral, ineffectual substance), while the capsules for the other group contained an antibiotic (doxycycline). All the capsules, identical in appearance, were prepared and "randomized" by the New York Hospital's pharmacy, which kept the identification codes sealed until this stage of the experiment was over. Thus, we had a more credible, double-blind trial; that is, neither we, the conductors of the experiment, nor the subjects knew at the time who had been given the placebo and who had been given the antibiotic.

At the end of the second month, the codes were opened, and the antibiotic was administered to those individuals who had been taking the placebo. This group went through another month of the same protocol. During each month of the experiment (two months for the women who had initially received the antibiotic, three months for the women who had initially received the placebo), all subjects were tested in the laboratory at appropriate points in their menstrual cycle for hormonal levels and bacteria. All subjects also participated in a six-month follow-up, which consisted of keeping a record of an entire menstrual cycle as a final evaluation document and imposing upon themselves the same restrictions that had applied earlier.

The bottom-line information we gained from this experiment is extremely heartening. At the end of the second month, we discovered that those women who had taken the antibiotic had experienced a dramatic improvement in their PMS symptoms while those who had taken the placebo had displayed no significant changes. After switching to doxycycline for the third month of the experiment, the former placebo takers registered the same high degree of improvement as their counterparts had. Six months later, a survey of all thirty subjects reported greatly reduced PMS difficulties across the board.

Three years following the conclusion of the therapy, I managed to interview twenty of our original subjects. Seven of these individuals enjoyed permanent improvement and were practically free of PMS symptoms. Unfortunately, the other thirteen gradually developed certain PMS symptoms, if not the full-blown syndrome, all over again. When I discussed our newer intravenous antibiotic treatment regimen, five of the thirteen reported for treatment courses. A look at the bacteriological isolates from these five patients revealed only anaerobic organisms from the initial culture studies—organisms on which doxycycline does not have a full-spectrum effect.

After concluding intravenous clindamycin and gentamicin courses, all five women responded with marked improvement in their PMS symptoms. Four of these women have so far remained symptom-free. One of them has remained symptom-free following a second course of the clindamycin and gentamicin intravenous treatment.

PMS continues to be a mystery inviting new theories and new treatment approaches. Mild sufferers get some relief from experimenting with self-help programs that include a restricted diet (frequent, small meals low in salt, sugar, caffeine, and alcohol), regular exercise, and ongoing stress-management techniques. Most serious sufferers, however, require medical assistance to overcome their symptoms.

Some doctors today advise altering the brain chemistry with "mood" or "diet" drugs, but this takes care of only those symptoms that are emotional in nature. Other doctors favor stopping ovulation altogether with drugs or surgery (usually by removing the ovaries, but sometimes by performing a hysterectomy). Obviously, this engineered end of menstruation means the end of PMS, but at a drastic price.

The 1987 study conducted at my laboratory does not, by any means, solve the mystery of PMS once and for all, but it does point to a promising new era in which PMS treatment for some women may not have to be so makeshift or hazardous. In the first place, the study suggests that the underlying cause of troublesome PMS symptoms in a significant number of patients may, indeed, be bacterial infection. Among the thirty subjects in the study, an unexpectedly high percentage of their endometrial biopsy cultures yielded positive findings for chlamydia, mycoplasma, and/or anaerobic bacteria. In the second place, the study suggests that low-risk, highly controllable antibiotic treatment is able to reverse troublesome PMS symptoms permanently.

Now, in the day-to-day activities of many of those women

who participated in the study, freedom from their PMS symptoms translates into greater comfort, enhanced pleasure, and improved productivity. What gratifies me even more, however, is that antibiotic therapy revived their healthy pelvic function.

PELVIC INFLAMMATORY
.... DISEASE ....

Like premenstrual syndrome, pelvic inflammatory disease (PID) is a clinical catchall title for an ill-defined malady. There is no symptom that clearly indicates the beginning of the illness, nor is there any certainty regarding what factors might turn a mild, subclinical condition into a clinically manifested, destructive process.

By strict definition, PID refers to any inflammation inside the pelvic cavity; thus, from a physiological standpoint, illnesses such as vaginitis, cervicitis, endometritis, salpingitis, and oophoritis are mere subcategories of PID. In medical practice, however, the diagnosis PID is reserved for relatively severe inflammations of the upper reproductive tract: the uterus, the fallopian tubes, and the ovaries.

PID is almost always set into motion by STDs—chief among them chlamydia and anaerobic bacterial infections. It is especially prevalent among women who first began having sexual intercourse at an early age, who have a history of multiple sexual partners, or who have relied on IUDs for birth control. The fact that IUD users are seven to ten times more likely to develop PID than women using barrier-type birth control methods is a strong indicator that PID is inclined to result from exposure to a male partner's seminal fluid during sexual intercourse.

In the typical PID case, harmful bacteria enter the upper part of the female genital tract, and the subsequent infection makes it easier for the native bacterial flora to proliferate and intensify the damage. Spermatozoa serve as an important vector in bacterial transfer. In those rare cases when a sexually abstinent woman develops PID, it is presumably because infectious bacteria—acquired during prior, sexually active years or via vertical transmission—have ascended through her genital tract during menstruation. In even rarer cases, bacteria from organs adjacent to the reproductive tract (such as the appendix or the bowels) can trigger a PID-causing infection.

As the most widespread and serious complication of sexually transmitted diseases, PID today is a medical and public health problem of rapidly escalating proportions. Experts claim that more than one million American women experience palpable symptoms of PID each year. Assuming 50 percent of all PID cases are asymptomatic, the number of actual PID victims would be twice as high. At least one third of the documented PID patients are eventually rendered infertile, and in 1989 alone (the last year for which estimates are available), the cost of treating PID and its consequences in the United States totaled over three billion dollars.

Much more worrisome than the monetary cost of PID is its cost in human misery. The typical PID symptom is mild lower abdominal discomfort or tenderness, but in bad cases, the pain grows noticeably worse over several days, perhaps becoming so strong that the victim has difficulty walking, urinating, or doing much else beyond merely enduring. At this point, treatment is mandatory. Otherwise, the infection could breed an abscess, which might burst and send life-threatening, infectious pus throughout the woman's abdominal cavity.

One night last year, Nora entered a local hospital emergency room with acute pain all across her abdomen and an enlarged mass on the left side of her pelvis. The initial interview revealed that she had been sexually active with one man for the last four months, had not used birth control, and had engaged in unusually strenuous sexual intercourse immediately before being taken to the emergency room by her partner.

Since Nora's vital signs were stable and she showed only a slight temperature, the problem was diagnosed and treated as a ruptured ovarian cyst. The attending doctor assumed the swelling in her pelvis was caused by blood. She spent a week in the hospital and was released.

I wound up taking over Nora's case shortly after her hospital stay, when her only complaint was a "slight tenderness in the abdomen or stomach, nothing much." Right from the start, I suspected her troubles were due to PID, not simply a ruptured ovarian cyst, and so I requested a sonogram. It confirmed my suspicion. One of her fallopian tubes was widely dilated and full of pus. Her ovary was swollen and full of cysts.

During the brief period of time involved in taking and interpreting the sonogram, Nora's pain steadily increased. Within a week, she developed a slight fever and, again, a small swelling in her pelvis that seemed to be caused by a fluid of some sort. Meanwhile, I analyzed her bacteria culture and found large amounts of chlamydia.

Nora's culture results, coupled with her latest symptoms, convinced me she was suffering from an advanced case of PID and that the fluid in her pelvis was due to the inflammation. I put her on a six-week doxycycline/erythromycin regimen and treated her partner with the same medication. She became symptom-free halfway into this therapy, and the results of her subsequent pelvic cultures were negative.

In Nora's case, a well-informed and well-conducted initial interview may have established the cause of her problem earlier, thus saving her a great deal of pain, time, trouble, and expense. The case of Sandy illustrates how proper history taking can aid a doctor in making a timely diagnosis of PID. I was on call for the hospital one night when the chief resident summoned me to give an opinion about a woman who had just been admitted to the emergency room and was in her twenty-fourth week of pregnancy. Surgical colleagues had already seen Sandy, had diagnosed tenderness in the area of her appendix and had recommended surgical exploration and a possible appendectomy. They wanted my input concerning the advisability of immediate surgery.

When I arrived at the hospital, the operating room had been fully prepared, and Sandy was ready to be taken upstairs for surgery. Simply approaching her from a distance, I observed that her midsection was much smaller than one would expect at the twenty-fourth week of a pregnancy. I couldn't help thinking that perhaps implantation had occurred in an already contaminated uterus, and now the fetus, deprived of nutrients, was lagging behind in development.

I proceeded to question her even before examining the lower right quadrant of her abdomen (where the appendix lies). As it turned out, this was Sandy's third pregnancy. The first one had taken place a few years back and had been interrupted after only six weeks. When we started discussing the second pregnancy, which had resulted in the birth of a boy, I chose my questions carefully to elicit possible evidence that the second pregnancy had taken place in a contaminated uterus.

"Was your son born either a few weeks prematurely or a few weeks late?" I asked.

"Yes," Sandy replied. "He was born six weeks before his due date."

Next I asked, "Am I correct in assuming that your son was born at a lower birth weight than you anticipated, even considering his prematurity?" Sandy's answer was again affirmative.

I went on to ask questions relating to the health of Sandy's son. Much to her amazement, I was right in my conjectures. Yes, her son was asthmatic. Yes, he had chronic ear infections. Yes, he had had a tonsillectomy at an early age.

At this point, I suspected that both the difficulties associated with the child's birth and his subsequent health problems could be traced to a contaminated uterine cavity. Most likely, the contamination had originally occurred at the time of Sandy's first pregnancy or shortly thereafter.

Then I asked Sandy's husband, Jack, whether he noticed any change in Sandy's personality after the birth of their son. "Yes, indeed!" Jack answered. "Not only was she more moody in general, but she'd throw tantrums every now and then, usually right before her period. We almost split up a couple of times because of these tantrums."

Sandy confirmed what Jack told me. When I asked her if there were any observable changes in her menstrual flow after giving birth, she nodded. "Before, my period used to last six or seven days," she recalled, "and there was a lot of bright, red blood. Afterward, it dwindled down to just a couple of days, with hardly any blood at all."

I was now convinced Sandy's current pregnancy was conceived in a highly unfavorable environment, where an ample number of bacteria were ready to cause a serious infection, given the opportunity. The pregnancy gave the bacteria that opportunity. The tenderness in her abdomen, I thought to myself, was not due to an inflamed appendix but to an infected fallopian tube. Turning to a nearby resident, who was obviously confused by the nature and meaning of my questions, I said, "Please cancel the surgery and call the chief resident."

When the chief resident came to the telephone, I told her I believed Sandy's problem was pelvic inflammatory disease—specifically, salpingitis. Rather than surgical intervention, I advised overnight intravenous administration of cefoxitin, a broad-spectrum antibiotic that would be perfectly safe for Sandy and her unborn child at this stage of the pregnancy. After a short argument, the chief resident consented to implement this course of treatment if I would take full responsibility.

About four days later, I met the chief resident in a hospital hallway. When I inquired about the follow-up to Sandy's antibiotic treatment, she said, "Well, after four more days of intravenous erythromycin, we discharged the patient, symptom-free."

"Why erythromycin?" I asked.

"The morning after she was admitted," the chief resident replied, "we got a positive confirmation of chlamydial infection in the patient's cervix." Thus, my hypothesis of PID due to bacterial infection was confirmed, and luckily for Sandy, no unnecessary surgery took place.

Sandy's case well illustrates the value of taking time to ask a patient questions. This common-sense but often overlooked strategy can lead to a much more accurate diagnosis, even before the results of laboratory work are available. Sandy's case also exemplifies the importance of exploring every possible avenue of questioning instead of leaping to conclusions. Despite the fact that pregnancy is rarely associated with such a dramatic flare-up of PID, the possibility cannot be ignored.

In the absence of gross symptoms like the ones Nora and Sandy exhibited, it is not always possible to detect the presence of PID in a woman's reproductive system. Even assuming medical science could do so, it is not practical to test on a routine basis every suspected high-risk individual. The cost to the patient—financially, physically, and emotionally—of performing a laparoscopy and culturing tissue samples is prohibitive.

The answer to this dilemma for millions of specific individuals and for public health in general lies in a more concerted effort to recognize, avoid, and solve reproductive health problems before they become so threatening. In the next chapter, I'll consider possible ways of making this important effort.

Chapter 6

....

Breaking the Circle:
The Fertile Future

To use a very appropriate metaphor, antibiotic therapy for reproductive health problems is still in its infancy. The child is growing and gathering strength, but it's too young to stand on its own. It continues to need a great deal of support, attention, and development. Assuming it prospers as it should, I believe it will be an exceptional gift to the world—one that holds the promise of breaking a vicious circle of pain, poor health, and infertility now being passed from one generation to another as well as from one sexual partner to another.

Fifteen years ago, I was just beginning to prescribe antibiotics for the treatment of mycoplasmal infections, and I was virtually alone in doing so. At that time, routine testing procedures for chlamydia or anaerobic bacteria didn't even exist. Medical science has come a long way since then. Now virtually all fertility specialists who request my consultation in a case include the request for culture studies for mycoplasma, chlamydia, and anaerobic bacteria in their patient's work-up, and follow my recommended antibiotic regimen in treating organisms that my experience has shown to be harmful to the reproductive process.

Nevertheless, there remain many mysteries about bacteria and bacterial infection that need to be solved. And there remains the challenge of ensuring that all culture studies meet the same standards of thoroughness and reliability and that all treatments for bacterial infection are sufficiently far-reaching and powerful.

Whatever direction the medical community takes in fostering the effective growth of antibiotic therapy, it is only one of two "parents." The other parent is the nonmedical population. Breaking the circle of problems I've described in this book requires that people in general take it upon themselves to become better informed about reproductive health issues, particularly about the damage bacterial infections can cause, and that they assume more responsibility for maintaining their own well-being. This responsibility includes getting tested for bacteria and, if appropriate, conscientiously completing antibiotic therapy.

To a certain extent, the advent of AIDS in recent years has helped alert people to the potential dangers of careless sexual relations. No longer are most sexually active adults quite so willing or able to wait for a palpable problem to develop before they think about reproductive health care. More men use condoms. More women insist their male partners use condoms. More couples avoid intercourse altogether until some degree of mutual commitment has been made.

Unfortunately, concern about AIDS has also had an adverse impact on popular attitudes toward responsible reproductive health practices. Many people so deeply mourn the demise of the "free sex" atmosphere associated with the 1960s and 1970s that they idealize promiscuity. They feel AIDS is the only barrier to sexual freedom, but in doing so they forget the many other dangers of irresponsible sex. Such public attitudes keep us from paying more attention to the seriousness of such STDs as bacterial infection.

Another problematic outcome of the current focus on AIDS is that health conditions not perceived as immediately life threatening tend to be ignored. Few realize bacterial infection can, in fact, lead to an early death. Considering that the government and other funding institutions are so slow to finance research into a disease as horrifying as AIDS, it is little wonder they are even slower to provide grants for the study of "lesser" reproductive health problems, such as those caused by bacteria.

Ideally, I would like the federal government to declare bacterial infection in the reproductive system a major public health issue and to authorize, say, five billion dollars to facilitate appropriate research and therapy. This sum is approximately equal to the sum this country will pay in a few years' time for treating pelvic inflammatory disease and its most serious complication, ectopic pregnancies. It does not come close, however, to including the total cost of infertility-reversing procedures.

For a few moments, let's assume my dream comes true. What research needs to be done? What therapeutic programs should be implemented?

ANTIBIOTIC THERAPY:
.... RESEARCH CHALLENGES ....

Often my patients—or nonmedical people who have heard about my work—say to me, "Antibiotic therapy for reproductive health problems is so simple and so effective, and it makes so much sense. Why doesn't every doctor or clinic offer it?" The only answer I can give them is that conventional approaches to health care are slow to change in the absence of repeated scientific proof that a change is warranted.

For all its success in short-term, double-blind studies and in the laboratory of human experience, the type of antibiotic therapy I advocate is still new and, therefore, still in the process of proving itself. We know antibiotic therapy works, but until we know more about how and why it works, it will continue to be categorized as an experimental therapy.

How, then, would I allocate the research half of my hypothetical five-billion-dollar federal grant? What specific research goals do I feel most need to be met in order to make antibiotic therapy for reproductive health problems universally accepted, available, and even mandatory in certain situations?

First, we must design studies that will yield a more precise identification and characterization of every type of bacteria that can be found in the human reproductive system. At present we can only single out a small percentage of bacteria that by association are suspected of causing reduced fertility or interference with the course of the pregnancy and the health of the newborn. In time, I believe we will find that many more are implicated.

A detailed mapping should be made to identify the bacterial flora present in the genital tracts of truly fertile couples (i.e., apparently harmless bacteria) and the bacterial flora present in the genital tracts of those couples who experience infertility or troubled pregnancies (i.e., apparently harmful bacteria). For each harmful bacterium we find, we must establish clear answers to two basic questions: What is its autogenic (that is, self-generated) role? What kind of immune response does it elicit?

After obtaining the answers to these questions, we can proceed to the second important phase of research: studying each bacterium in reference to its involvement in specific reproductive health problems. These problems are the ones I've described in earlier chapters of this book: localized infections, hormonal imbalances, functional interference in the genital tract, miscarriages, and so on.

Right now, following strict scientific standards, we can make only an anecdotal connection between bacteria and many of these problems. We can say, for example, "Fran had a chlamydia infection, and later, she miscarried." But what, exactly, was the physiological nature of the link between these two facts? Why did the chlamydia in Fran's system evolve beyond being a mere opportunistic cohabitant to become an outright pathogen? Did it function in concert with other types of bacteria in her system? What else was happening in her system during the same period of time? Did any of these events contribute to the infection or the miscarriage?

The results of this second phase of research will establish scientific proof that bacteria do, indeed, have a cause-and-effect role in the development of reproductive health problems. Without such a scientific basis, antibiotic therapy for such problems can't be institutionalized, however successful the therapy may be in practice. And without institutionalization, there will continue to be a dearth of testing centers technologically sophisticated enough to isolate harmful bacteria—a situation that currently imposes a severe limit on the potential widespread use of antibiotic therapy.

Unfortunately, research into bacterial infections in the reproductive system and their response to antibiotic therapy can never be conducted according to the rigid clinical standards that apply to most other forms of medical research. These standards include completing double-blind studies (studies during which neither the volunteers nor the administrators know who's taking a placebo) at least two years in length. It would be inhumane to ask infertility patients—especially women who are in their late thirties or early forties—to remain on a placebo for two years. Under the circumstances, I believe most scientists will accept considerably shorter studies, as long as they are otherwise well designed and well implemented.

Of course, many reproductive health specialists have already become enthusiastic prescribers of antibiotic therapy. They have been converted to this therapy by the positive results of dozens of short-term, double-blind studies conducted over the past ten years within the medical system (that is, in the context of clinical research, which is not as strict as academic research). Among these studies has been the six-month, PMS-related study I supervised in 1986 (see Chapter 5). In the future, we must have repeated proof of these studies, as well as new studies altogether to confirm what we now only suspect and to uncover what now lies beyond our suspicions.

ANTIBIOTIC THERAPY:
.... A PREVENTIVE APPROACH ....

Once science verifies and articulates the major role played by bacteria in triggering reproductive health problems, the human race can enter into an exciting new era of reproductive health care. Today, the type of broad-spectrum antibiotic therapy I recommend for my patients is relatively unknown. Even if it were better known, most testing centers are ill equipped to facilitate it, and most doctors are not trained to take adequate patient histories in order to detect possible bacterial infections. As a consequence, when antibiotic therapy is administered these days, it's usually to treat diseases and maladies that have already caused considerable damage. In the future, when antibiotic therapy has gained widespread acceptance and availability, it can be aimed mainly at preventing diseases and malfunctions before they ever have a chance to develop.

In essence, the prophylactic prevention of bacterially related reproductive health problems requires the administration of different antibiotic treatment regimens at different periods in every individual's life. Specifically, bacterial testing would become routine procedure for both males and females at birth, at puberty, prior to marriage, and prior to attempting a pregnancy (women would also be routinely tested after giving birth). In addition, bacterial testing would be a standard procedure whenever an individual experienced any genital-tract pain or problem. If such testing revealed the presence of harmful bacteria, then the appropriate course of antibiotic treatment would be given.

At this point, let us review those symptoms or circumstances that I believe would indicate the possible presence of harmful bacteria in a patient's genital tract at the time of his or her birth. Chief among such symptoms and circumstances are:

- A premature or postdated pregnancy

- Early rupture of the amniotic membranes

- The existence of an intrauterine infection in the mother during pregnancy

- A pregnancy complicated by toxemia or preeclampsia

- An intrauterine infection called chorioamnionitis

143

- A low birth weight or growth retardation, especially when inflammation of the placenta can be histologically documented

- Severe postpartum infection in the mother, particularly endometritis

- The only-child syndrome, when it can be established that secondary infertility in the mother may have had an infectious origin, in which case the harmful bacteria were probably present in her system before she gave birth to her only child

- Conception soon after a miscarriage, without the mother having been properly treated with antibiotics

Besides these warning signals, I also think doctors in the future will suspect possible bacterial infection whenever they encounter a patient whose mother delivered by cesarean section. In my opinion, the great majority of cesarean sections not indicated by a genuine size discrepancy between the mother and the infant may be performed either because the uterus failed to respond to natural hormonal stimulation or because the labor contractions were too strong to enable a poorly implanted placenta to supply the infant with oxygen during the delivery process. Both of these conditions could be due to bacterial infection in the mother's uterine lining prior to implantation.

In the future, doctors will probably also be suspicious of a lengthy labor in their patient's birth history. Bacteria in the mother might have compromised the myometrial contractibility. In such a situation, the infant is worse off passing through an infected birth canal after the protective membranes are broken than being delivered by cesarean section. In my own practice to date, I've had to reverse my originally negative attitude toward cesarean section because I realized it often has the potential of rescuing a baby from the serious bacterial contamination that could result if he or she were left inside the mother during a lengthy labor. I have also become more and more convinced that it is prudent to treat an intrauterine baby exposed to potential infection during the course of the pregnancy itself. Since the early 1980s, I have managed patients who were in early premature labor with antibiotics: orally at first; later, intravenously. The side effects of these antibiotics for the baby are negligible; and the fact that pregnancies so treated go to term even after membranes have ruptured testifies to the value of such management.

Any of the above-mentioned indicators of possible bacterial infection at the time of a patient's birth should warrant immediate bacterial testing. Should the presence of potential pathogens become apparent, case-appropriate antibiotic treatment should be given. Ideally this testing and treatment will occur as soon after a patient's birth as possible.

Because the pediatric community at present does not officially accept that genital-tract infections can be vertically transmitted, there is no body of information that would enable me to project whether any bacterial testing or antibiotic treatment for children is likely to become a part of future reproductive health care. The need to develop this information through research is urgent. For all we know at this point, it may be possible for bacteria to multiply and turn destructive in an individual's genital tract even before puberty or before any history of sexual intercourse. In a female child, bacteria may be proved capable of ascending to the ovaries; in a male child, to the epithelium in the testes.

If periodic medical intervention—perhaps at milestones in a

child's physical development—could detect such dangers and prevent them from happening, then it should become routine. Of course, now as well as in the future, if a child actually exhibits any symptoms of trouble in the genital tract, bacterial testing and, possibly, antibiotic treatment are definitely advisable.

Assuming there are no relevant problems after a child's birth, the next routine testing for bacterial infection should occur at puberty, while the patient is still a virgin. As discussed in previous chapters, hormonal changes associated with puberty can, I believe, suddenly spur the growth of vertically transmitted bacteria that have lain dormant in the individual's genital tract up until that stage of his or her life. A female victim of such bacterial growth may remain asymptomatic, or she may develop menorrhagia, dysmenorrhea, vaginitis, and/or a host of ovarian-cystic conditions. A male victim may also remain asymptomatic, or he may develop urethritis and/or prostatitis.

In my ideal future, for all women during and after puberty, bacterial testing would be added to the routine gynecological testings most clinics now offer. For all men during and after puberty, semen analysis in general, including bacterial testing, would become routine for the first time in history.

Exactly how routine bacterial testing should be in an individual adult's life—that is, how often he or she needs to be tested—is conjectural right now, pending further research. Based on what we do know so far, a bacteria-free adult who is celibate shouldn't need frequent bacterial testing; nor should a bacteria-free adult who has a monogamous relationship with a bacteria-free partner. A sexually active adult with multiple partners, however, should be tested whenever he or she changes partners (the optimum situation, of course, is for both new partners to be tested together). As I've already mentioned, I would advise making culture testing for bacteria—followed, if applicable, by antibiotic treatment—a prerequisite for a marriage license.

Once during a public interview I was asked if I would condone the routine administration of (for example) a three-week Vibramycin course prior to an attempted conception for any couple living in a geographical area where testing procedures are not readily available. My unequivocal answer was, "Yes!" In fact, I would probably give this regimen in combination with erythromycin or Flagyl for a five- to six-week duration. Having worked with these antibiotics for the last decade, I know that their side effects are insignificant and are capable of being tolerated with only minor discomfort. Until the time when testing procedures are universally offered and available, I believe that routine pre-conceptional antibiotic therapy would prevent innumberable miscarriages or troubled pregnancies. Speaking for myself as a doctor in such a situation, I am quite willing to take the blame for administering antibiotics without thorough testing when the potential return is so precious.

In my dream scenario of the future, I would also like to see bacterial testing and treatment become a routine first-step procedure in preconception child planning and an early follow-up procedure for women after giving birth. Although it would be difficult to make these procedures mandatory, they could be tied to hospital admission and discharge. Better yet, they could become standard practice in a whole new network of pregnancy clinics that would evolve to facilitate every stage of a pregnancy from a couple's first intention to reproduce to the final postpartum care of the mother and newborn.

My notion of pregnancy clinics in the future is not at all farfetched. Obstetrics today, which technically confines itself to the actual delivery of a child, is turning into an increasingly high-risk profession. More and more, we're learning that many complications with which an obstetrician must deal, including the ones we've examined in this book, are predetermined at conception or even earlier. Given the rising rate of problem pregnancies, the litigious nature of our society, and the distorted expectation among many would-be parents that modern technology can guarantee perfect babies, obstetricians today must pay exorbitant malpractice-insurance premiums. I project the escalating bacterial contamination of the general population is bound to bring all these matters to a head very soon, provoking major alterations in how medical specialists define their responsibilities and how medical care is extended to prospective parents and their babies.

THE ANTIBIOTIC FUTURE:
.... POSSIBLE IMPLICATIONS ....

The timetable for personal bacterial testing and treatment I have just outlined, along with the establishment of pregnancy clinics, promises to create stronger bridges among different existing fertility therapies. For example, I predict bacterial testing and treatment will become an integral part of in vitro fertilization. In my own laboratory, where the two therapies are already linked, it is an enormous joy to help a woman who has been through numerous unsuccessful in vitro cycles finally achieve an in vitro pregnancy after a two-week clindamycin and gentamicin course. I also believe future research will demonstrate that bacterial infections initiate infertility problems in the immune system; thus, bacterial testing and treatment will merge with immunological fertility therapy.

Because it stretches across a patient's life span, the timetable I've outlined strongly suggests that antibiotic therapy to maintain reproductive health will become a multidisciplinary option. As individuals go through different physical and emotional changes and consult different kinds of specialists, they will repeatedly encounter the possible prescription of bacterial testing and antibiotic therapy. It will be a treatment regimen associated with pediatrics, gerontology, and even psychiatry as well as gynecology, obstetrics, and urology.

The institutionalization of bacterial testing and antibiotic therapy could also have profound side effects on the attitudes and behaviors of the general population. Knowing how infectious bacteria are spread and how to prevent their spread, individuals may become more circumspect in their sexual lives, in their choice of marriage partners, and in their approach to family planning. In the future, potential parents will not only strive to achieve a particular pregnancy but will also have the utmost concern for maintaining their genital-tract purity, in order to allow themselves the freedom to reproduce at will.

Tricky ethical issues may arise. For example, infected people who are unable to reproduce may be able to sue the partners who infected them. A new component may have to be added to rape cases, since the rapist may actually transmit an infection to his victim that renders her infertile. Publicity campaigns to encourage cooperation with reproductive health programs may have to be launched and ways found to persuade individuals and groups to engage in socially responsible sexual and reproductive conduct.

Even the most vigorous efforts, however, are bound to fall short of the goal of entirely eradicating reproductive bacterial infection from the population. Some people will continue to be troubled by infection-related fertility problems. Thus, couples considering the termination of a pregnancy through abortion—particularly if it is the woman's first pregnancy—may want to take this factor into account when making their decision. Because bacterial infection compromises fertility in a progressive manner, first pregnancies often produce the healthiest offspring. Each successive pregnancy may yield weaker children, so the termination of any pregnancy may mean taking the chance that later pregnancies may be more difficult or produce less healthy children.

REPRODUCTIVE HEALTH:
.... WHAT YOU CAN DO NOW ....

Until reproductive health is recognized by the medical establishment and the federal government as a major public health issue, thereby ensuring better, more concerted efforts at research, consumer education, and consumer protection, infertile couples must make their own way through the vast, intimidating wilderness of fertility specialists and therapies. To make this quest less perilous, nothing is more important than information.

When a man and a woman suspect that they are suffering from infertility, the first thing they should do is read about infertility on their own. Fortunately, many widely available books offer comprehensive and reliable basic information on infertility and are written in layperson's language. My advice is to read several of these books and make notes.

However fast-paced recent scientific developments in the field of infertility have been, the major tests and treatments have not changed much, and they're likely to remain the same for years to come. The more you learn about these tests and treatments—why they are prescribed, how they are administered, and what the results may be—the more potentially successful your campaign to overcome infertility will be. You will be able to talk more constructively with fertility specialists, develop more reasonable expectations regarding what different therapies can do for you, and cooperate more effectively in giving specific therapies their best chance of working.

When you feel you are fairly well informed about the different types of fertility specialists and what they do, then gather as much information as you can about the specialists who practice in your area. Consult friends and local professional groups for recommendations, and interview several specialists before making a final decision about which one to retain. It will cost money to shop around in this manner, but it will be money very well spent, given what a mistake in judgment may cost you.

The relationship between an infertility patient and a fertility specialist is uniquely intimate, requiring a great deal of mutual trust and respect. It makes far more sense to spend time and money up front finding the best specialist for your physical and emotional needs than to waste time and money over several months or even years on a specialist who ultimately proves to be inappropriate.

Here, to get you started, are some sources of information regarding infertility and fertility specialists:

- American College of Obstetricians and Gynecologists
  Resource Center
  409 Twelfth Street, SW, Washington, DC 20024
  (202) 638-5577
  National professional organization for obstetricians and
  gynecologists; offers printed materials regarding reproductive
  health and infertility plus information about contacting obstetricians and gynecologists across the nation

- American Fertility Society
  2140 Eleventh Avenue, South, Suite 200, Birmingham, AL
  35205
  (205) 933-8494
  National organization of fertility specialists; offers printed
  materials regarding infertility

- American Urological Association
  1120 North Charles Street, Baltimore, MD 21201
  (301) 727-1100
  Offers printed materials regarding urology and male reproductive health plus information about contacting urologists
  across the nation

- Planned Parenthood Federation of America
  810 Seventh Avenue, New York, NY 10019
  (212) 541-7800
  Offers information about contacting affiliated groups across
  the nation, which can supply information about local fertility
  specialists, clinics, and resource centers

- Resolve, Inc.
  5 Water Street, Arlington, MA 02174
  (800) 662-1016/(617) 643-2424

Self-help organization for infertile couples; offers printed materials regarding infertility plus information about contacting affiliated groups across the nation, which can supply information about local fertility specialists, clinics, resource centers, and support groups

As a general rule for choosing a specialist, I would suggest going to a large fertility clinic. There, you will find a number of specialists whom you may interview, all of whom have had the benefit of each other's counsel and quality control.

I particularly recommend fertility clinics affiliated with teaching institutions. Because of the very active communication and loan network among teaching institutions, their fertility clinics are most likely to utilize the very latest information, instruments, and techniques in their therapies.

Before or during your initial interview of a specialist, here are some very basic questions to which you need answers:

- In what areas of medicine is the specialist certified: obstetrics and gynecology, urology, reproductive endocrinology?

- What specific reproductive health problems does the specialist treat?

- What tests, procedures, medications, and treatments does the specialist offer? What is the average total cost and total time span of different types of therapies?

- How many patients has the specialist treated? What is the specialist's overall rate of success for different therapies (interpreted as the percentage of live births among the total number of couples treated)?

- With what types of patients does the specialist usually work? What, for example, is the average age of the specialist's patients?

- Does the specialist personally handle all aspects of a patient's case?

- Who else may become involved in a patient's case? What are the qualifications of that individual (or those individuals)? What might be the extent of such involvement?

- Is the specialist readily available for consultation? Are there certain times of the day or days of the week that the specialist is more (or less) likely to be available?

- How does the specialist handle the patient's insurance?

Some answers may immediately disqualify particular specialists. For example, they may not offer services that you want, or their prices may be too high. Other answers may not mean much to you because you don't yet know enough about your particular infertility problem to interpret their relevance. Nevertheless, it's critical to get all the advance information you can so you can monitor progress in your case and anticipate possible problems, alternatives, and needs.

Be sure to pose the same questions to each specialist you interview. This will give you a more accurate basis for comparing one with another. And it's in the context of such a comparison that many of the individual answers you've accumulated will acquire more significance.

Above all, pay attention to how sensitively and thoroughly each specialist frames his or her responses. Try to assess whether one specialist inspires your confidence more than any of the others, or whether he or she seems to have a more knowledgeable approach to infertility problems or an approach that is more compatible with your own ideas and feelings.

Once you finally decide upon a specialist, make sure at all times during your doctor-patient relationship that you have a clear sense of how your case is progressing and some idea of what to expect a month down the line, three months down the line, a year down the line. Your specialist should provide you with a systematic plan for making progress in treating your infertility. If such a plan is lacking or if your patience is exhausted, then you should seek help elsewhere. For all you know, you may be dealing with someone who has, in fact, quite legitimately run out of ideas. Remember it's never too late to get a second opinion or change specialists if you feel you're in a rut—for example, repeating the same therapy over and over, always experiencing the same type of failure, and never having a reason to believe the future holds anything different. I offer only one cautionary note, for those patients who have been treated for infectious bacteria with antibiotics. It is good to keep in mind that the period of greatest fertility following a negative culture study is *not* the following month. As several months pass by, the individual's fertility improves; and it may be approximately six to ten months before optimal restoration of the reproductive process is achieved, provided there is no pre-treatment structural damage. The explanation for this time lag is probably the fact that once bacterial infections are eliminated, the immune system requires time to restore the local environment to normal.

Before you change specialists, it's critical to get all the information you can about your case from the specialist you're leaving. Insist upon receiving copies of every test the specialist has performed, and check to see that these copies are dated and include all relevant information. Such documents are extremely helpful to any future specialist you may consult and can save you a great deal of time, money, and frustration.

BRINGING ABOUT THE
·········· FERTILE FUTURE ··········

Just as infertile couples critically need information, the field of infertility treatment critically needs informed consumers. Today, too much energy is expended on reversing or overcoming problems that may never have materialized in the first place if the patients presenting the problems had been more enlightened about, and responsible for, their own reproductive health. The more effort an individual can contribute to his or her own well-being, the more effort medical science can devote to making progress on promising treatment breakthroughs like antibiotic therapy.

When infertility problems or other reproductive health problems do arise, informed patients can save their specialists, not to mention themselves, a great deal of time if they already have a good, general background knowledge relative to their situation. They can also make far more intelligent choices among the specific treatment options they are offered.

The future of antibiotic therapy for reproductive health problems hinges on the public's becoming more aware of why that therapy is so promising and on individual patients' actively seeking that therapy from their specialists. Left to its own devices, without the watchdog influence or intelligent decision making of an informed public, institutionalized reproductive health care has pretty much confined itself to the treatment of outright infertility—a very advanced reproductive health problem—and has become relatively fixated on complex, high-risk, and expensive assisted-reproduction technologies (like in vitro fertilization) that try to work around infertility problems instead of correcting them.

I believe we need to identify and attack reproductive health problems much earlier, much more directly, and much less dangerously than we do now. Most important of all, I believe we need to identify and attack reproductive health problems more successfully than we do now. I am convinced antibiotic therapy has the capacity to satisfy all these needs.

It is, indeed, possible that the near future will bring about substantial government support for antibiotic therapy and that the general population will have the information and the means to live much healthier lives and produce much healthier offspring. If this support doesn't materialize, it is highly probable that the near future will at least bring about laws to curb escalating reproductive health care costs and educate the public about such preventive reproductive health strategies as bacterial testing and antibiotic treatment. What is absolutely certain is that the near future will bring about increasing public discussion of reproductive health care in general and antibiotic therapy in particular. We owe that discussion to the next generation—and to every generation that follows.

Glossary

Abortion: a premature ending of a pregnancy that is either induced or spontaneous (i.e., a miscarriage).

Adhesion: scar tissue that develops on the site of an infection, inflammation, or surgical incision and that can prevent normal egg or sperm passage and/or interfere with zygote implantation.

Amenorrhea: the absence of menstruation.

Anaerobic Bacteria: a type of bacteria that can survive in an oxygen-poor environment. In the genital tract, some kinds of anaerobic bacteria can cause infections that may lead to infertility.

Artificial Insemination (AI): the insertion of a sperm sample inside the female genital tract by artificial means. "Donor insemination (AID)" refers to sperm from a man other than the woman's partner.

Asymptomatic: exhibiting no symptoms.

Bacteria: single-celled living organisms, some of which can trigger infections in the reproductive system.

Basal Body Temperature (BBT): the lowest body temperature during the day (usually early morning). For a woman, the BBT has a pattern of being lower than normal prior to ovulation and higher than normal after ovulation.

Biopsy: a small sample of body tissue removed for microscopic examination.

Capacitation: the process of preparing sperm by artificial means so that their chances of fertilizing an egg are enhanced.

Cervix: the tube-like lowermost portion of the uterus that opens into the vagina. "Cervicitis" refers to inflammation of the cervix.

Chlamydia: a kind of bacteria that is responsible for infections of the genital tract, especially through sexual transmission.

Chlomiphene: a fertility drug (marketed as Clomid or Serophene) that stimulates ovulation.

Corpus Luteum: literally, a "yellow body" that forms in the ovary on the site where an egg has been released and that produces progesterone to facilitate a pregnancy.

Diethylstilbestrol (DES): a synthetic estrogen, taken by women in the past to prevent miscarriages, that has been associated with infertility and other reproductive health problems in some male and female offspring.

Dilation and Curettage (D&C): an operation in which the cervix is stretched to permit scraping of the uterine lining.

Ectopic Pregnancy: a pregnancy that takes place outside of its normal location, the uterus. Ectopic pregnancies most often occur in a fallopian tube.

Egg: the female reproductive cell, also called an "ovum" or "oocyte."

Embryo: the fertilized egg after it has divided and until the end of its second month of development.

Embryo Transfer: the process of taking an embryo that has developed in vitro and placing it in the uterus for implantation and further development.

Endometrium: the lining of the uterus that swells after ovulation to receive an egg and is sloughed off during menstruation if implantation doesn't take place. "Endometritis" refers to inflammation of the endometrium. "Endometriosis" refers to growth of the endometrium outside the uterus, which can result in damage to the reproductive system and, possibly, infertility.

Epididymis: a thin, coiled, tube-like structure through which sperm travel from the testicles to the vas deferens. "Epididymitis" refers to inflammation of the epididymis.

Estrogen: a female sex hormone that stimulates egg and endometrium development prior to fertilization.

Fallopian Tube: a narrow duct (there are two in the female genital tract) that receives the egg from the ovary, and in which the egg and the sperm meet for fertilization. "Salpingitis" refers to inflammation of the fallopian tube.

Fertilization: the union of the sperm with the egg in the fallopian tube, representing the initial step in a pregnancy.

Fetus: the unborn baby from its second month of development until its birth.

Fibroid Tumor: a tumor in the uterus that may interfere with pregnancy.

Gamete: a reproductive cell, either egg or sperm.

Gamete Intrafallopian Transfer (GIFT): a surgical process whereby eggs and sperm are put together outside of the woman's body and then placed inside her fallopian tube for fertilization to occur.

Human Chorionic Gonadotropin (HCG): female hormone that stimulates ovulation (often injected as a fertility drug).

Hysterosalpingogram: an X-ray examination of the uterus and the fallopian tubes.

Hysteroscopy: an examination of the uterus by means of a thin instrument inserted through the cervix.

Intratubal Insemination (ITI): artificial insemination in which the sperm are placed into the fallopian tubes instead of the vagina (the most common target of artificial insemination).

Intrauterine Insemination (IUI): artificial insemination in which the sperm are placed into the uterus.

In Vitro Fertilization: fertilization outside the body ("in vitro" is Latin for "in a glass").

Karyotyping: a test that analyzes chromosomes to determine if there is a genetic basis for repeated miscarriages.

Laparoscopy: a surgical procedure in which a thin, telescope-like instrument is inserted into the abdominal cavity to visualize or repair reproductive health problems.

Luteal Phase: the postovulation phase of the menstrual cycle. "Luteal phase defect" refers to the inadequate production of hormones during this phase to support a pregnancy.

Menarche: the time when a woman has her first menstruation.

Menopause: the time when a woman ceases to menstruate for natural, age-related reasons.

Microsurgery: surgery performed on the genital tract using microscopic instruments under magnification.

Miscarriage: a spontaneous abortion, or termination, of a pregnancy.

Mycoplasma: a type of bacteria that can cause infections in the genital tract.

Oligospermia: a low sperm count.

Ovary: the female gonad (there are two ovaries in the female genital tract) that produces eggs and hormones. "Oophoritis" refers to inflammation of the ovary.

Pelvic Inflammatory Disease (PID): an infection occurring in the female reproductive system, of which vaginitis, cervicitis, salpingitis, and oophoritis are subsets.

Pergonal: a fertility drug used to induce ovulation.

Postcoital Test: a test performed on cervical mucus a few hours after intercourse to determine the number and motility of sperm.

Progesterone: a female hormone produced by the ovary that prepares the uterine lining for egg implantation.

Semen: fluid containing the sperm and nourishing secretions that is expelled from the male reproductive system by means of ejaculation.

Sexually Transmitted Disease (STD): a reproductive health problem attributable to an infectious agent passed from one partner to another during sexual intercourse.

Sperm: the male reproductive cell. "Sperm antibodies" refers to agents in the man's or woman's body fluids produced by the immune system that reduce fertility by harming or killing sperm. "Sperm count" refers to the number of sperm in an ejaculate. "Sperm motility" refers to the movement capabilities of individual sperm. "Sperm morphology" refers to the structure of individual sperm.

Split-Ejaculate: seminal fluid with an enhanced concentration of sperm created by splitting an ejaculated semen sample (the first half of the ejaculate contains most of the sperm).

Superovulation: the production of multiple eggs during a single menstrual cycle stimulated by fertility drugs.

Testicles: the male gonad (there are two testicles in the male genital tract) that produces sperm and hormones.

Testosterone: the primary male sex hormone that contributes to sperm production.

Ultrasound: a technique of visualizing the interior of the body, including the genital tract, using sound-wave emissions.

Ureaplasma: the smallest known member of the mycoplasma family.

Uterus: the womb.

Vagina: the "birth canal" leading from the vulva to the cervix. "Vaginitis" refers to inflammation of the vagina.

Varicocele: an enlarged vein in the scrotum that can lead to infertility.

Vas Deferens: the tube through which sperm pass from the epididymis to the urethra. "Vasectomy" refers to a surgical sterilization of this tube.

Zona Pellucida: the protective surface layer of the egg.

Zygote: a fertilized egg that has not yet divided.

Zygote Intrafallopian Transfer (ZIFT): in vitro fertilization that involves creating a zygote outside the body and then placing it into the fallopian tube.

Index

Vagina, 48
  acidic milieu, 82
  irritation of the, 111
Vaginitis, 40, 48, 50, 63, 65,
    91, 116, 118–21, 127,
    146
Varicocele, 26, 40, 88–93
Vas deferens, 26
Venereal disease, *see* Sexually
    transmitted diseases

Vertical transmission of bacterial
    infection, 36, 52–60, 113, 120,
    128, 145, 146
  symptoms of, 62–63
Vibramycin, 13, 147
Vibra-Tabs, 54
Viruses, 29

Yeast infections, *see* Vaginitis
Yeasts, 29